Rehabilitation in Developing Countries

Editor

JOSEPH P. JACOB

PHYSICAL MEDICINE AND REHABILITATION CLINICS OF NORTH AMERICA

www.pmr.theclinics.com

Consulting Editor
SANTOS F. MARTINEZ

November 2019 • Volume 30 • Number 4

ELSEVIER

1600 John F. Kennedy Boulevard ● Suite 1800 ● Philadelphia, Pennsylvania, 19103-2899

http://www.theclinics.com

PHYSICAL MEDICINE AND REHABILITATION CLINICS OF NORTH AMERICA Volume 30, Number 4
November 2019 ISSN 1047-9651, ISBN 978-0-323-71044-2

Editor: Lauren Boyle
Developmental Editor: Laura Fisher

Reprints. For copies of 100 or more of articles in this publication, please contact the Commercial Reprints Department, Elsevier Inc., 360 Park Avenue South, New York, NY 10010-1710. Tel.: 212-633-3874; Fax: 212-633-3820; E-mail: reprints@elsevier.com.

Physical Medicine and Rehabilitation Clinics of North America (ISSN 1047-9651) is published quarterly by Elsevier Inc., 360 Park Avenue South, New York, NY 10010-1710. Months of issue are February, May, August, and November. Business and Editorial Offices: 1600 John F. Kennedy Blvd., Suite 1800, Philadelphia, PA 19103-2899. Customer Service Office: 3251 Riverport Lane, Maryland Heights, MO 63043. Periodicals postage paid at New York, NY and additional mailing offices. Subscription price per year is $304.00 (US individuals), $600.00 (US institutions), $100.00 (US students), $366.00 (Canadian individuals), $790.00 (Canadian institutions), $210.00 (Canadian students), $429.00 (foreign individuals), $790.00 (foreign institutions), and $210.00 (foreign students). Foreign air speed delivery is included in all *Clinics* subscription prices. All prices are subject to change without notice. **POSTMASTER:** Send address changes to *Physical Medicine and Rehabilitation Clinics of North America*, Customer Service Office: Elsevier Health Sciences Division, Subscription Customer Service, 3251 Riverport Lane, Maryland Heights, MO 63043. **Customer Service: 1-800-654-2452 (US). From outside of the United States, call 314-447-8871. Fax: 314-447-8029. E-mail: JournalsCustomer Service-usa@elsevier.com (for print support); JournalsOnlineSupport-usa@elsevier.com (for online support).**

Physical Medicine and Rehabilitation Clinics of North America is indexed in *Excerpta Medica, MEDLINE/ PubMed (Index Medicus), Cinahl,* and *Cumulative Index to Nursing and Allied Health Literature.*

Contributors

CONSULTING EDITOR

SANTOS F. MARTINEZ, MD, MS
Diplomate of the American Academy of Physical Medicine and Rehabilitation, Certificate of Added Qualification Sports Medicine, Assistant Professor, Department of Orthopaedics, Campbell Clinic Orthopaedics, University of Tennessee, Memphis, Tennessee, USA

EDITOR

JOSEPH P. JACOB, MD
Physiatrist, UCHealth, Fellow, American Academy of Physical Medicine and Rehabilitation, UCHealth Physical Medicine and Rehabilitation Clinic, Loveland, Colorado, USA

AUTHORS

BADRUNNESA AHMED, MBBS, FCPS
Associate Professor, Department of Physical Medicine and Rehabilitation, Bangabandhu Sheikh Mujib Medical University, Dhaka, Bangladesh

SYED MOZAFFAR AHMED, MBBS, FCPS
Professor, Department of Physical Medicine and Rehabilitation, Bangabandhu Sheikh Mujib Medical University, Dhaka, Bangladesh

CHULHYUN AHN, MD, MS
Clinical Assistant Professor, Department of Physical Medicine and Rehabilitation, Geisinger Health System, Danville, Pennsylvania, USA

BHASKER AMATYA, DMedSc, MD, MPH
Senior Project Manager, Department of Rehabilitation, Royal Melbourne Hospital, Research Coordinator, Australian Rehabilitation Research Centre, Honorary Fellow, Department of Medicine, University of Melbourne, Parkville, Victoria, Australia

TESFAYE BERHE ASEGAHEGN, MD
Associate Professor (Neurology), PMR Fellow, Department of Neurology, St Paul's Hospital Millennium Medical College, Addis Ababa, Ethiopia

LINAMARA RIZZO BATTISTELLA, MD, PhD
Full Professor of Physical Medicine and Rehabilitation, University of Sao Paulo, School of Medicine, Chair of Lucy Montoro Rehabilitation Medicine Institute, Clinical Hospital of USP, Sao Paulo, Brazil

GRACIELA BORELLI, MD
Profesora Agregada de Rehabilitación y Medicina Física, Cátedra de Rehabilitación, Universidad de la República, Montevideo, Uruguay

NATHAN BRAY, PhD
School of Health Sciences, Bangor University, Bangor, Gwynedd, United Kingdom

ASARE B. CHRISTIAN, MD, MPH
Outpatient Medical Director, Good Shepherd Rehabilitation Hospital, Allentown, Pennsylvania, USA

SILVANA CONTEPOMI, PT
Asociación Argentina de Tecnología Asistiva (AATA), San Isidro, Argentina

SANDRA CORLETTO, MD
Directora, Especialista en Medicina Física y Rehabilitación, Especialista en Neurodiagnóstico, Centro de Rehabilitación y Electrodiagnostico CRE, Honduras

WOUTER DE GROOTE, MD, PRM
Postgraduate Rehabilitation Management in the Global South, Chair ISPRM-WHO "Rehabilitation Capacity Building in LMIC"; Rehabilitation Department, AZ Rivierenland, Bornem, Belgium

MARIA HERRERA DEAN, MD
Médico Fisiatra, Gerente centro Especializado de Medicina Fisica y Rehabilitación, Instituto Hondureño de Seguridad Social, San Pedro Sula, Honduras

RAJU DHAKAL, MBBS, MD
Medical Director, Physical Medicine and Rehabilitation, Spinal Injury Rehabilitation Centre, Sanga, Nepal

MARY P. DOHERTY, RTR
Vice President, Hackett Hemwall Patterson Foundation, Madison, Wisconsin, USA

MOHAMMAD ALI EMRAN, MBBS, FCPS
Associate Professor, Department of Physical Medicine and Rehabilitation, Bangabandhu Sheikh Mujib Medical University, Dhaka, Bangladesh

JULIA PATRICK ENGKASAN, MBBS, MRehab Med, PhD
Associate Professor, Consultant Rehabilitation Physician, Department of Rehabilitation Medicine, Faculty of Medicine, University of Malaya, Kuala Lumpur, Malaysia

MAELU FLECK, BS
Executive Director, American Association of Orthopaedic Medicine, Ridgeway, Colorado, USA

SISAY GIZAW GEBEREMICHAEL, MD
Assistant Professor (Neurology), PMR Fellow, Department of Neurology, St Paul's Hospital Millennium Medical College, Addis Ababa, Ethiopia

MARY GOLDBERG, PhD
International Society of Wheelchair Professionals, Department of Rehabilitation Science and Technology, Human Engineering Research Laboratories, University of Pittsburgh, Pittsburgh, Pennsylvania, USA

JAMES GOSNEY, MD, MPH
Resident Physician, Department of Physical Medicine and Rehabilitation, Geisinger Health System, Danville, Pennsylvania, USA

CHRISTINE C. GROVES, MD
Physical Medicine and Rehabilitation, Spinal Injury Rehabilitation Centre, Sanga, Nepal;
Department of Physical Medicine and Rehabilitation, Indiana University School of
Medicine, Indianapolis, Indiana, USA

JORGE GUTIÉRREZ, MD
Centro de Rehabilitación Potenciales, Cali Valle, Colombia

JUAN MANUEL GUZMÀN, MD
Academic, Professor and Chair, Physical Medicine and Rehabilitation, Electrodiagnostic
and EMG, Mexican Academy of Surgery, Mexico City, Mexico

ANDREW J. HAIG, MD
Professor Emeritus, The University of Michigan, Ann Arbor, Michigan, USA; President,
Haig Consulting PLC, Michigan, USA

NAZIRAH HASNAN, MBBS, MRehab Med, PhD
Associate Professor, Consultant Rehabilitation Physician, Department of
Rehabilitation Medicine, Faculty of Medicine, University of Malaya, Kuala Lumpur,
Malaysia

OHNMAR HTWE, MBBS, MMedSc (Rehab Med), CMIA
Associate Professor, Consultant Rehabilitation Physician, Rehabilitation Medicine Unit,
Department of Orthopedics and Traumatology, Faculty of Medicine, University
Kebangsaan Malaysia, Kuala Lumpur, Malaysia

MARTA IMAMURA, MD
Departamento de Medicina Legal, Etica Medica e Medicina Social e do
Trabalho, Faculdade de Medicina FMUSP, Universidade de Sao Paulo, Sao Paulo,
Brazil

MOHAMMAD TARIQUL ISLAM, MBBS, FCPS
Associate Professor, Department of Physical Medicine and Rehabilitation, Bangabandhu
Sheikh Mujib Medical University, Dhaka, Bangladesh

MRINAL JOSHI, MBBS, MD, DNB, MNAMS, GCMskMed
Director and Professor, Rehabilitation Research Center, SMS Medical College and
Hospitals, Jaipur, India

PADMAJA KANKIPATI, PhD
Specialized Mobility Operations & Innovation, Bangalore, India

FARY KHAN, MBBS, MD, FAFRM (RACP)
Director, Department of Rehabilitation, Royal Melbourne Hospital, Clinical Director,
Australian Rehabilitation Research Centre, Clinical Professor, Department of Medicine,
Adjunct Professor, Disability Inclusive Unit, Nossal Institute of Global Health, University of
Melbourne, Parkville, Victoria, Australia; Adjunct Professor, School of Public Health and
Preventative Medicine, Monash University, Clayton, Victoria, Australia

MOHAMMAD MONIRUZZAMAN KHAN, MBBS, FCPS
Professor, Department of Physical Medicine and Rehabilitation, Bangabandhu Sheikh
Mujib Medical University, Dhaka, Bangladesh

MOHAMMAD NURUZZAMAN KHANDOKER, MBBS, FCPS
Associate Professor, Department of Physical Medicine and Rehabilitation, Bangabandhu
Sheikh Mujib Medical University, Dhaka, Bangladesh

MOSHIUR RAHMAN KHASRU, MBBS, FCPS
Associate Professor, Department of Physical Medicine and Rehabilitation, Bangabandhu Sheikh Mujib Medical University, Dhaka, Bangladesh

SU YI LEE, MBBS, FAFRM (RACP)
Rehabilitation Specialist, Department of Rehabilitation, Royal Melbourne Hospital, Research Fellow, Australian Rehabilitation Research Centre, PhD Candidate, Department of Medicine, University of Melbourne, Parkville, Victoria, Australia

JIANAN LI, MD
Chief, Medical Rehabilitation Center, Nanjing Medical University, Nanjing, China

LEONARD S.W. LI, MBBS, FRCP, FAFRM(RACP), FHKAM(Medicine)
Director, Neurological Rehabilitation Centre, Virtus Medical Center, Honorary Clinical Professor, Department of Medicine, University of Hong Kong, Hong Kong SAR, China

MAZLINA MAZLAN, MBBS, MRehab Med, CMIA
Associate Professor and Consultant Rehabilitation Physician, Department of Rehabilitation Medicine, Faculty of Medicine, University of Malaya, Kuala Lumpur, Malaysia

WILLIAM MICHEO, MD
Professor and Chair, Director, Sports Medicine Fellowship, Physical Medicine, Rehabilitation and Sports Medicine Department, University of Puerto Rico, School of Medicine, San Juan, Puerto Rico, USA

MOHAMMAD MOYEENUZZAMAN, MBBS, FCPS
Professor, Department of Physical Medicine and Rehabilitation, Bangabandhu Sheikh Mujib Medical University, Dhaka, Bangladesh

DIANA MUZIO, MD
Jefe de servicio de Fisiatria del Instituto de Reahabilitacion Psicofisica, Profesora a Cargo de la Carrera Universitaria de Medicina Física y Rehabilitación, Médica Fisiatra de FLENI, Directora de Centro de Rehabilitación CRIA, Universidad de Medicina de Buenos Aires, Buenos Aires, Argentina

SHAMSUN NAHAR, MBBS, FCPS
Professor, Department of Physical Medicine and Rehabilitation, Bangabandhu Sheikh Mujib Medical University, Dhaka, Bangladesh

AMARAMALAR SELVI NAICKER, MBBS, MRehab Med, CIME
Professor and Consultant Rehabilitation Physician, Rehabilitation Medicine Unit, Department of Orthopedics and Traumatology, Faculty of Medicine, University Kebangsaan Malaysia, Kuala Lumpur, Malaysia

MANIMALAR SELVI NAICKER, MBBS, MPath, MMedStats
Lecturer and Consultant, Department of Pathology, Faculty of Medicine, University of Malaya, Kuala Lumpur, Malaysia

BRYAN O'YOUNG, MD
Physical Medicine and Rehabilitation Residency Program Director, Department of Physical Medicine and Rehabilitation, Geisinger Health System, Danville, Pennsylvania, USA; Clinical Professor, New York University School of Medicine, New York, New York, USA

DAVID RABAGO, MD
Associate Professor, Department of Family Medicine and Community Health, University of Wisconsin School of Medicine and Public Health, Madison, Wisconsin, USA

MAHMUDUR RAHMAN, MBBS, FCPS
Associate Professor, Department of Physical Medicine and Rehabilitation, Bangabandhu Sheikh Mujib Medical University, Dhaka, Bangladesh

MOHAMMAD HABIBUR RAHMAN, MBBS, FCPS
Professor, Department of Physical Medicine and Rehabilitation, National Institute of Traumatology, Dhaka, Bangladesh

MOHAMMAD SHAHIDUR RAHMAN, MBBS, FCPS
Professor, Department of Physical Medicine and Rehabilitation, Bangabandhu Sheikh Mujib Medical University, Dhaka, Bangladesh

KENNETH DEAN REEVES, MD, FAAPM&R
Private Practice, Physical Medicine and Rehabilitation, Roeland Park, Kansas, USA

ABUL KHAIR MOHAMMAD SALEK, MBBS, FCPS
Professor, Department of Physical Medicine and Rehabilitation, Bangabandhu Sheikh Mujib Medical University, Dhaka, Bangladesh

CAROLINA SCHIAPPACASSE, MD
Head of Rehabilitation Department, British Hospital, Directora, Clínica de Rehabilitación Las Araucarias, Professor of Biomechanics, San Martin University, Buenos Aires, Argentina

MOHAMMAD ABDUS SHAKOOR, MBBS, FCPS, PhD
Professor, Department of Physical Medicine and Rehabilitation, Bangabandhu Sheikh Mujib Medical University, Dhaka, Bangladesh

FARZANA KHAN SHOMA, MBBS, FCPS
Assistant Professor, Department of Physical Medicine and Rehabilitation, Bangabandhu Sheikh Mujib Medical University, Dhaka, Bangladesh

ABENA YEBOAA TANNOR, BSc, MBChB, MSc (Rehab), MGCP
Sports, Exercise and Rehabilitation Medicine Fellow, Specialist Family Physician, Department of Family Medicine, Family Medicine Directorate, Adjunct Lecturer, Disability and Rehabilitation Studies, Komfo Anokye Teaching Hospital, Kwame Nkrumah University of Science and Technology, Kumasi, Ghana

GEORGE THARION, MBBS, DPMR, D Ortho, DNB(PMR), MD(PMR)
Professor, Department of Physical Medicine and Rehabilitation, CMC Vellore, Vellore, Tamil Nadu, India

RAJI THOMAS, MBBS, DPMR, MD(PMR), DNB(PMR)
Professor and Head, Department of Physical Medicine and Rehabilitation, CMC Vellore, Vellore, Tamil Nadu, India

MARÍA LUISA TORO-HERNÁNDEZ, PhD
School of Physiotherapy, Universidad CES, Medellín, Colombia

DENISE RODRIGUES TSUKIMOTO, OT
Physical Medicine and Rehabilitation Institute (IMREA), Hospital das Clinicas, University of Sao Paulo, Sao Paulo, Sao Paulo, Brazil

TASLIM UDDIN, MBBS, FCPS
Professor and Chairman, Department of Physical Medicine and Rehabilitation,
Bangabandhu Sheikh Mujib Medical University, Dhaka, Bangladesh

MOHAMMAD AHSAN ULLAH, MBBS, FCPS
Professor, Department of Physical Medicine and Rehabilitation, Bangabandhu Sheikh
Mujib Medical University, Dhaka, Bangladesh

VANDANA VASUDEVAN, MBBS, FAFRM (RACP)
Rehabilitation Specialist, Department of Rehabilitation, Royal Melbourne Hospital,
Research Fellow, Australian Rehabilitation Research Centre, Parkville, Victoria, Australia

GLORIA VERGARA-DIAZ, MD
Research Fellow, Department of Physical Medicine and Rehabilitation, Harvard Medical
School, Spaulding Rehabilitation Hospital, Boston, Massachusetts, USA

SAARI MOHAMAD YATIM, MD, MRehab Med
Consultant Rehabilitation Physician, Department of Rehabilitation Medicine, Hospital
Serdang, Selangor, Malaysia

BRENDA SARIA YULIAWIRATMAN, MBBS, MRehab Med, CMIA
Rehabilitation Physician, Rehabilitation Medicine Unit, Department of Orthopedics and
Traumatology, Faculty of Medicine, University Kebangsaan Malaysia, Kuala Lumpur,
Malaysia

YUSNIZA MOHD. YUSOF, MBBS, MRehab Med
Consultant Rehabilitation Physician, Department of Rehabilitation Medicine, Hospital
Rehabilitasi Cheras, Kuala Lumpur, Malaysia

Contents

A profound need for rehabilitation services exists, particularly in developing countries. This article highlights the role of the epidemiology of disability in addressing this critical need. It aims to: (1) introduce the concepts of "disability" and "functioning" based on the WHO International Classification of Functioning, Disability and Health (ICF); (2) address disability measurement methodology generally to include common national and international methodologies; (3) highlight specific relevant 2017 Global Burden of Disease (GBD) results; (4) profile current global demographic trends of disability related to non-communicable diseases and the aging population, and; (5) provide disability considerations for health and human rights.

Community-based rehabilitation (CBR) has changed considerably over 4 decades, resulting in a rights-based approach, holding local authorities accountable for service delivery. For medical rehabilitation in low-resource countries, there is concern about how this service gap will be covered. The CBR community continues to strengthen the evidence base for CBR implementation, acknowledging its extensiveness and variety on the ground. The creation of standardizing tools favors this process because it provides the building blocks to scale up, setting standards for implementation research. Finally, an International Classification of Functioning, Disability, and Health–based assessment and intervention model for CBR is proposed.

Rehabilitation plays a crucial role in natural disasters owing to the significant upsurge of survivors with complex and long-term disabling injuries. Rehabilitation professionals can minimize mortality, decrease disability, and improve clinical outcomes and participation. In disaster-prone countries, skilled rehabilitation workforce and services are either limited and/

or comprehensive rehabilitation-inclusive disaster management plans are yet to be developed. The World Health Organization Emergency Medical Team initiative and guidelines provide structure and standardization to prepare, plan, and provide effective and coordinated care during disasters. Many challenges remain for implementation of these standards in disaster settings and integrating rehabilitation personnel.

Chronic musculoskeletal pain and disability dramatically reduce quality and
quantity of life worldwide, disproportionately so in low- and middle-income
countries. Complementary therapies not typically learned in conventional medical training have much to offer but are under-utilized. Prolotherapy is an
injection-based complementary therapy supported by high-quality evidence
for osteoarthritis, tendinopathy, and low back pain. Prolotherapy addresses
causes of pain and disability at the tissue level, is straightforward to learn,
and relies on common, inexpensive material, and requires no refrigeration.
Not-for-profit organizations are delivering prolotherapy to underserved patients in low- and middle-income countries through service-learning projects.

As a low-income country with a significant burden of disease and frequent
natural disasters, the need for rehabilitation in Nepal is significant. Rehabilitation services currently available in Nepal are limited, but the government
has recently adopted a 10-year action plan to address rehabilitation needs
nationwide. Rehabilitation education and training is necessary to provide
and retain adequate multidisciplinary rehabilitation providers for current
and future needs in Nepal. The implementation of evidence-based recommendations to improve the quality of rehabilitation services and access to
rehabilitation is critical to maximize individual and community well-being.

Physical rehabilitation medicine started in Bangladesh 50 years ago, but
there is no documentary evidence stating its origin, history of progression
as a specialty, and work with agenda items. A gap exists between
disability-related health and participation, which affects service delivery
systems offered to persons with disability (PwD). Disability prevalence
ranges from 0.47% to 14.4%. Illiteracy, maldistribution of wealth, and
increasing prevalence of chronic diseases add to the burden of existing
disability. It is necessary to involve all stakeholders in disability management to strengthen medical rehabilitation teams and improve service delivery while advocating for the rights and needs of PwD.

This article reviews the epidemiology, rehabilitation intervention strategies,
and rehabilitation resources for persons with disabilities (PWD) in

Malaysia. Currently, the registered number of PWD is 409,269 individuals, 1.3% of the total population, which is far less than the World Health Organization estimation of 10%. The rehabilitation implementation strategies include health policies, health promotion, and prevention programs. Health-related services for PWD are provided by many government agencies, including health, welfare, education, manpower, housing, and the private sector and nongovernment organizations. It is hoped national health programs can ensure special care and rehabilitation for PWD, optimizing self-reliance and social integration.

Raji Thomas and George Tharion

The article describes the rehabilitation services provided at Christian Medical College Vellore, a tertiary care medical college hospital in South India. The department was started by Dr Mary Verghese, who on completion of her medical training sustained spinal cord Injury with resulting paraplegia. Following a section on the initial beginnings of the department, the current status of the department offering comprehensive rehabilitation by the multidisciplinary team is highlighted. The article ends with the challenges faced, including limitations in providing affordable solutions, architectural and attitudinal barriers, and inadequate number of rehabilitation physicians and comprehensive rehabilitation centers in the country.

Mrinal Joshi

Earlier rehabilitation interventions, like community-based rehabilitation (CBR), could not make a remarkable impact because they ran parallel to the health system, but the newer model establishes health-related rehabilitation as an integral part of the health care system at all levels and thus should be implemented as such. Collaborating with other players relevant to the CBR matrix, such as social and vocational services, can be imparted for the empowerment of a disabled group at the village level through the CBR center. A multipurpose rehabilitation worker, through skill transfer or task shifting, can start rehabilitation at the primary health center.

María Luisa Toro-Hernández, Padmaja Kankipati, Mary Goldberg, Silvana Contepomi, Denise Rodrigues Tsukimoto, and Nathan Bray

Access to appropriate and affordable assistive technology is a human right, and a public health and development priority. This article elaborates on these aspects and illustrates the various opportunities and barriers to achieving equitable access to assistive technology through 4 specific country snapshots. In Brazil, mobility aids are provided through universal health coverage in rehabilitation reference centers in urban areas. A community-based rehabilitation pilot project in Argentina demonstrates how to reach an excluded indigenous community. A rapidly developing national legal framework in Colombia with imminent implementation challenges is showcased, as is a technology transfer model in India.

An increase in population and chronic conditions leading to disability require increasing emphasis on rehabilitation and health intervention. Poorer countries do not usually have the rehabilitation workforce needed to promote societal inclusion and participation. The roles of the rehabilitation workforce were often not clearly defined, leading to task shifting among rehabilitation professionals. Barriers to capacity building were poor availability of human resources and insufficient training program/supports for their professional development. Facilitators were local government support and international non-governmental organizations collaboration. Recommendations for capacity building effort are for collaboration with the developed nations to encourage funding, training, education, and sharing of resources.

PHYSICAL MEDICINE AND REHABILITATION CLINICS OF NORTH AMERICA

FORTHCOMING ISSUES

February 2020
Cerebral Palsy
Aloysia L. Schwabe, *Editor*

May 2020
Pharmacologic Support in Pain Management
Steven Stanos and James R. Babington, *Editors*

August 2020
Spinal Cord Injury
John L. Lin, *Editor*

RECENT ISSUES

August 2019
Medical Impairment, Disability Evaluation and Associated Medicolegal Issues
Robert D. Rondinelli and Marjorie Eskay-Auerbach, *Editors*

May 2019
Technological Advances in Rehabilitation
Joel Stein and Leroy R. Lindsay, *Editors*

February 2019
Polytrauma Rehabilitation
Blessen C. Eapen and David X. Cifu, *Editors*

SERIES OF RELATED INTEREST

Orthopedic Clinics
Clinics in Sports Medicine

VISIT THE CLINICS ONLINE!
Access your subscription at:
www.theclinics.com

Foreword
A Call to Arms

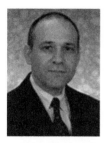

Santos F. Martinez, MD, MS
Consulting Editor

The degree to which a disability limits one's acceptance and ability to function in society varies. Despite ingenuity and fortitude, factors such as material and financial resources, access to adequately trained professionals, and cultural heterogeneity need to be considered. Fortunately, there are numerous national and international organizations dedicated to this mission in developing countries. Such gallant efforts and dialogue can make a considerable difference to countless individuals who, otherwise, would be destined to much less tolerable conditions.

It is hoped that Dr Jacob's interests, efforts, and success in producing this common-ground issue for sharing ideas will cultivate ongoing alliances. The Physiatrist along with the aid of like-minded subspecialties (Physical Therapy, Occupational Therapy, Speech Therapy, Prosthetics/Orthotics, Psychology, and so on) can facilitate this undertaking. We encourage those who sense this calling to become actively engaged to share their talents and energy with this very worthwhile endeavor.

Santos F. Martinez, MD, MS
American Academy of Physical Medicine
and Rehabilitation
Campbell Clinic Orthopaedics
Department of Orthopaedics
University of Tennessee
Memphis, TN 38104, USA

E-mail address:
smartinez@campbellclinic.com

Phys Med Rehabil Clin N Am 30 (2019) xv
https://doi.org/10.1016/j.pmr.2019.08.003
1047-9651/19/© 2019 Published by Elsevier Inc.

pmr.theclinics.com

Preface

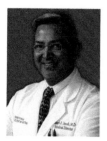

Joseph P. Jacob, MD
Editor

Growing up in rural South India, I witnessed the lifelong effects of polio in my great-uncle and the effects of disability in my grandfather after he suffered a stroke. There were minimal access to health care of any type and no access to medical rehabilitation.

The epidemiology of disability in low-resource areas of the world varies from the developed world in terms of impairment categories as well as age groups affected.

There is limited awareness of the epidemiology of disability and available resources in low-resource areas of the world. The resources vary from community-based rehabilitation to specialized services provided in tertiary rehabilitation centers.

There is a need for locally relevant cost-effective service delivery models and technologies in low-resource regions. Insights from such models of delivery and technologies may also be relevant in improving services for the disabled in low-resource pockets of more advanced countries.

This issue of *Physical Medicine and Rehabilitation Clinics of North America* seeks to highlight local strategies for disability prevention, community-based rehabilitation, and development of innovative cost-efficient local delivery systems and technology.

I extend my thanks to the authors for their contributions to this issue and their ongoing efforts to advance the care of persons with disabilities in their communities.

Joseph P. Jacob, MD
UCHealth Physical Medicine and
Rehabilitation Clinic
2695 Rocky Mountain Avenue
Suite 200
Loveland, CO 80538, USA

E-mail address:
physicalrehabmd@gmail.com

Phys Med Rehabil Clin N Am 30 (2019) xvii
https://doi.org/10.1016/j.pmr.2019.08.002
1047-9651/19/© 2019 Published by Elsevier Inc.

pmr.theclinics.com

Introduction

Rehabilitation in developing countries has changed considerably over the years. Many activities were initiallly based on the charity model of care for people with a disability. In a later stage, with the introduction of community-based rehabilitation, the world got acquainted with the first concept of rehabilitation in an attempt to compensate for unavailable services, using peer support as the main mechanism for implementation.

Since then, many efforts have been made by low- and middle-income countries ranging from training and capacity building of rehabilitation staff, the establishment of procurement systems for assistive devices, the inclusion of rehabilitation activities in disaster relief programs, integration of rehabilitation clinics into health care systems as well as ratification of the UN Convention on the Rights of Persons with Disabilities.

Nevertheless, only 20% of the rehabilitation workforce resides in low- and middle-income countries. Alarmingly, in Sub-Saharan Africa, there are only a dozen Physical Medicine and Rehabilitation doctors, which contributes to the challenges in addressing rising rates of noncommunicable diseases.

In order to strengthen the capacity of rehabilitation further, a concerted action is key. We need end-users to advocate for inclusive policies and affordable services, academics to collaborate across national borders, ministries of health to strengthen the health care system for rehabilitation, international nongovernmental organizations need to continue raising awareness and contributing to sustainable measures, and international professional bodies need to build capacities of their counterparts. Most of all, ongoing change will come with local ambassadors for rehabilitation, who play a crucial role to inspire and keep pushing the agenda forward in their country.

In the long run, we want to attain Universal Health Coverage, which means that rehabilitation must be included in health system planning and strengthening. For low- and middle-income countries, whenever possible, special attention is required for the integration of rehabilitation services into the primary health care level: accessibility is a key component of service delivery in a context where access to services can be challenging due to geographic, transport, and financial constraints that can impede service engagement for the user.

Therefore, we are grateful for this issue of *Physical Medicine and Rehabilitation Clinics of North America* dedicated to "developing" countries. The reader is provided with updates from different regions all over the world. It is useful to learn from scientific data and the whereabouts of rehabilitation in many settings: it inspires, and it is hoped, cross-fertilizes with opportunities and good practices.

Wouter De Groote, MD, PRM
Rehabilitation Department
AZ Rivierenland
Kasteelstraat 23
Bornem 2880, Belgium

E-mail address:
Wouter.de.groote@telenet.be

Phys Med Rehabil Clin N Am 30 (2019) xix
https://doi.org/10.1016/j.pmr.2019.08.004
1047-9651/19/© 2019 Published by Elsevier Inc.

The Concept and Epidemiology of Disability

Bryan O'Young, MD[a,b,]*, James Gosney, MD, MPH[a], Chulhyun Ahn, MD, MS[a]

KEYWORDS

- Disability • Disability epidemiology • Disability measurement methodology
- Disability measurement instrument • Global disability rates
- Global burden of disease (GBD) • WHO International Classification of Functioning
- Disability and health (ICF)

KEY POINTS

- According to the World Health Organization International Classification of Functioning, Disability and Health, "disability" is an integrative concept that represents the negative interaction between an individual's health conditions and personal and environmental contextual factors.
- Common national disability measurement instruments include censuses and surveys. International methodologies that serve to standardize data comparison across countries, regions and populations are the WHO Disability Assessment Schedule (WHODAS 2.0) and the Global Burden of Diseases, Injuries, and Risk Factors Study 2017 (GBD 2017).
- GBD 2017 results show that the total burden of disability increased by 52% between 1990 and 2017. Low back pain, headache disorders, and depressive disorders were the leading causes of disability globally in 2017.
- Global disability rates are increasing due to increasing noncommunicable diseases and the aging population.

INTRODUCTION

The current model of "disability" has developed beyond the inceptual World Health Organization (WHO) International Classification of Impairment, Disability and Handicap (ICIDH; 1980), which primarily interpreted "disability" as a limitation in one's activity due to underlying body pathology and impairment. Today's WHO International Classification of Functioning, Disability and Health (ICF; 2001)–based model also considers the effect of environmental and personal factors on body functions, activity, and

Disclosure Statement: The authors have nothing to disclose.
[a] Department of Physical Medicine and Rehabilitation, Geisinger Health System, 100 North Academy Avenue, Danville, PA 17822, USA; [b] New York University School of Medicine, New York, NY 10067, USA
* Corresponding author. Department of Physical Medicine and Rehabilitation, Geisinger Health System, 100 North Academy Avenue, Danville, PA 17822, USA
E-mail address: boyoung1@geisinger.edu

Phys Med Rehabil Clin N Am 30 (2019) 697–707
https://doi.org/10.1016/j.pmr.2019.07.012
1047-9651/19/© 2019 Elsevier Inc. All rights reserved.

participation domains, which enables fuller measurement of health status. National and global efforts to measure health status and disability seek to quantify, clarify, and interpret these contributing factors and their relationships to influence public policy and design programs intended to positively impact the lives of anyone experiencing disability.

This article on the concept and epidemiology of disability for this special issue on rehabilitation in developing countries describes the concept of disability based on the ICF and preceding ICIDH, as well as how disability has evolved from a medical to a human rights construct. Disability measurement methodology is addressed generally, and relevant results of the 2017 Global Burden of Disease (GBD) study are highlighted. Current demographic trends of increasing disability due to noncommunicable diseases and the aging global population are noted. Pediatric demographics are addressed. The article continues with disability considerations regarding health, the environment, and human rights and socioeconomic inequality.

WHAT IS DISABILITY?

I lost my leg by landmine when I was 5 years old, at that time I went to the rice field with my mother to get firewood. Unfortunately I stepped on a mine. After the accident I was very sad when I saw the other children playing or swimming in the river because I have no leg. I used to stand with my crutch made of wood and I wish I could play freely like the other children too. And when I walked to school some children they called me kombot, meaning disabled person, and [the discrimination] make me feel shy and cry and disappointed. So I want all people to have equal rights and not discriminate against each other.

—*Song*

At the age of 9, I became deaf as a result of a bout with meningitis. In 2002, I went for Voluntary Counseling and Testing (VCT). The results showed that I was HIV+ [positive for human immunodeficiency virus]. I become devastated and lost hope to live because I thought that being HIV+ was the end of world for me. Later, I met a disabled person who spiritually encouraged me to accept my status. Now I have confidence to be able to speak out on HIV/AIDS openly. I have been interviewed widely by print and electronic media and I have been invited to speak in public meetings. I am creating awareness on the importance of VCT and encouraging people to know their status. My work is limited by lack of money. Deaf people living in rural areas have no information on HIV/AIDS. I would like to break the barriers by going to visit them right where they live.

—*Susan*

What makes me to feel not included in this school is because my parents are poor, they can't provide me with enough books. This makes my life difficult in the school. They also can't buy me everything which I am supposed to have, like clothes. Being in school without books and pens also makes me feel not included, because teachers used to send me out because I don't have books to write in.

—*Jackline*

Disability is a multifaceted, evolving, and contested concept. Language such as "handicapped worker" is now seldom used, nearly universally replaced by "disability-first" phraseology. Although blind and deaf persons and individuals in wheelchairs are stereotypes of persons with disability, health conditions associated with disability are varied and heterogeneous. They can be temporary, episodic, chronic, or progressive. Rather than be characterized by a normal-abnormal dichotomy, the concept of disability encompasses a continuum ranging from minor limitations in functioning to complete dependence for all daily activities of living.

Characterization of disability has shifted from a "medical model," whereby individuals were viewed as being disabled by their medical condition or impairment, to a "social model" that emphasizes environmental and societal components. The *Preamble* to the Convention on the Right of Persons with Disabilities (CRPD) addresses the social aspect of disability, indicating that "disability results from the interaction between persons with impairments and attitudinal and environmental barriers that hinder their full and effective participation in society on an equal basis with others,"[1] serving to help establish disability as a human rights issue.

Lack of a standardized universal concept of "disability" has posed a major barrier to conceptualization and development of the epidemiology of disability to include contributing health and environmental factors. This lack of standardization has thereby impeded development of rehabilitation interventions to prevent and mitigate these factors as well as measures required to maximize the functioning and quality of life of persons experiencing disability. Furthermore, the ambiguous concept and definition of "disability" compromises research comparisons of disabilities across intervention, time, and region.

The International Classification of Functioning, Disability and Health (ICF) is a framework endorsed by the WHO that measures health status and disability at both individual and population levels. It uses a "bio-psycho-social model" that incorporates the multidimensional aspects of disability, considering functioning and disability as a "dynamic interaction between health conditions and contextual factors, both personal and environmental." "Disability" in the ICF framework is an umbrella term that encompasses impairments, activity limitations, and participation restrictions. It denotes the "negative aspects of the interaction between an individual (with a health condition) and that individual's contextual factors (environmental and personal factors)." The profiles in the preceding introduction personify "disability." **Fig. 1** and **Box 1** schematize the interaction between ICF components of the ICF model and provide supporting definitions. **Fig. 2** demonstrates these model interactions in terms of spinal cord injury, a specific health condition.

The ICF is a second-generation framework that builds on the concept of disability proposed by the preceding WHO ICIDH model. The ICIDH hierarchical framework hypothesized a causal chain linking "pathology," "impairment," "disability," and "handicap."[2] "Disability" was interpreted as a limitation in one's activity due to underlying pathology and impairment. This definition did not fully consider the effect of environmental and personal factors on activity level, as does the later ICF (environmental factors were acknowledged but not classified in the ICIDH). Because of the lack of influence attributed to environmental factors and the inability to fully measure health status using the ICIDH's limiting definition of disability, among other reasons, the ICIDH began to be ignored by disability data users and was superseded by the ICF model.[3]

Functioning and disability for health conditions and injuries classified in the ICF is intended to be correlated with ICD (International Classification of Diseases) diagnoses to provide a full picture of health and functioning in a consistent and internationally comparable manner.[4] Although ICD provides diagnoses, additional information from ICF on functioning may facilitate health planning and management. ICD and ICF are complementary.[5]

DISABILITY AND HEALTH

A medical condition may be classified as "primary," "secondary," or "comorbid" depending on whether it is the primary cause of disability, derived from the primary condition, or independent of the primary condition. The medical condition that initiates

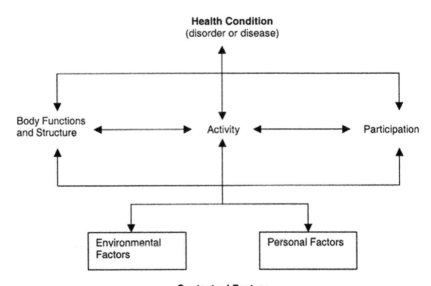

Contextual Factors

Fig. 1. The ICF model: the interaction between ICF components. (*From* World Health Organization. How to use the ICF: A practical manual for using the International Classification of Functioning, Disability and Health (ICF). Exposure draft for comment. Geneva: WHO; 2013. Available at: https://www.who.int/classifications/drafticfpracticalmanual.pdf; with permission.)

Box 1
Definitions of components of the International Classification of Functioning, Disability, and Health (ICF) model

Functioning is an umbrella term for body functions, body structures, activities, and participation. It denotes the positive aspects of the interaction between an individual (with a health condition) and that individual's contextual factors (environmental and personal factors).

Disability is an umbrella term for impairments, activity limitations, and participation restrictions. It denotes the negative aspects of the interaction between an individual (with a health condition) and that individual's contextual factors (environmental and personal factors).

Body functions: The physiologic functions of body systems (including psychological functions).

Body structures: Anatomic parts of the body, such as organs, limbs, and their components.

Impairments: Problems in body function and structure such as significant deviation or loss.

Activity: The execution of a task or action by an individual.

Participation: Involvement in a life situation.

Activity limitations: Difficulties an individual may have in executing activities.

Participation restrictions: The physical, social, and attitudinal environment in which people live and conduct their lives. These are either barriers to or facilitations of the person's functioning.

From World Health Organization. How to use the ICF: A practical manual for using the International Classification of Functioning, Disability and Health (ICF). Exposure draft for comment. Geneva: WHO; 2013. Available at: https://www.who.int/classifications/drafticfpracticalmanual.pdf; with permission.

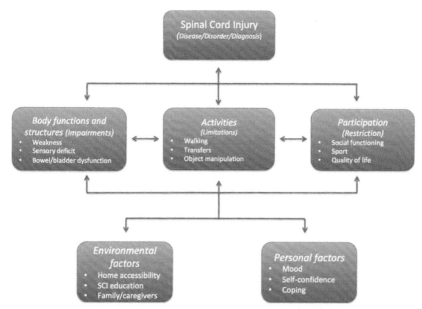

Fig. 2. Health condition of a patient with spinal cord injury (SCI).

impairment, activity limitation, or participation restriction is referred to as the "primary health condition."[6] Examples of primary health conditions include degenerative joint disease, amputation, cerebrovascular accident, chronic obstructive pulmonary disease, coronary artery disease, depression, and Duchenne muscular dystrophy. The primary health condition may result in a variety of impairments that can affect mobility, sensation, cognition, and communication.[6] Notwithstanding the primary health condition, however, individuals may enjoy good health. A person with impaired hearing may not have ongoing health care needs, for example.

A "secondary health condition" is an additional health condition that occurs due to the primary health condition and whose risk is increased by the presence of the primary condition. Examples of secondary conditions for spinal cord injury include heterotopic ossification, urinary tract infections, pressure injuries, and depression. Depression, pain, and osteoporosis are other common secondary conditions. Secondary conditions can decrease patient level of function and quality of life, as well as increase morbidity and mortality.[6]

Last, a "comorbid" condition is defined as an additional health condition that is unrelated to the primary condition. An example of a comorbid condition is diabetes in a blind individual. Comorbid conditions are often not well diagnosed or well managed.[7] The risks of certain chronic conditions are higher in people with mobility deficits.[8] Multiple comorbidities and secondary conditions are associated with more severe disability, which requires more complex health and rehabilitative care.[9]

MEASURING DISABILITY

Measurement of nonfatal loss of health is a significant epidemiologic challenge due to the development of new treatment methods, emergence of new diseases, and the increasing number of individuals globally who survive injuries and diseases but are left with health loss.[10] Data on impairment may only be an approximate surrogate measure of disability, as disability is based on an individual's difficulty in functioning in the context of his or her environment. Further, disability data may not be included in existing classification systems and in many countries data on rehabilitation are not disaggregated from other health care services.

Given that disability is a universal experience and a matter of degree, countries increasingly use a continuous scale to assess the level of disability. Estimates of the incidence and prevalence of disability differ based on thresholds for various domains of disability. National estimates of disability are also affected by the data collection instrument used. Censuses poll entire populations, but typically query a limited number of disability-related items and therefore tend to provide lower estimates of disability prevalence than do surveys. Data analyses in censuses are basic; questions are simply dichotomized and not analyzed with item response theory methods that would allow for development of a metric scale, for example. Moreover, censuses are responded to by the household head, which results in underreporting. However, regular censuses can trend disability over time. Surveys may yield more detailed information on the disability, including bodily impairment and function as well as individual activity and participation levels.

A comprehensive national disability monitoring system would include personal factors, such as somatic and psycho-cognitive impairments, functional limitations, and restrictions in participation, as well as environmental factors. Disability severity and duration should be measured for all age groups and living situations including group residential and institutional settings. Personal and environmental disability risk factors identified through monitoring can inform development of interventions to prevent and mitigate barriers to individual activity and participation in society.

Historically, variation of disability definitions and measurement methodologies across countries has challenged data collection of national relevance on an international scale.[6,11,12] Standardization of national disability measurement instruments results in improved data comparison across countries, regions, and populations. Data comparison can be achieved by use of a common framework for collection of individual data by an instrument such as the ICF, which uses a universal reporting coding system.[5] Implementation of the ICF at the population level includes health and disability data collection in surveys of general and specific populations, data compilation and analysis, and development of disability survey modules and question sets.[3] The ICF establishes domains of human functioning at the body, person, and society levels, and provides operational definitions of disability based on decrements in functioning domains.[5] Linked directly to the ICF via common usage of foundational concepts and definitions, the WHO Disability Assessment Schedule (WHODAS 2.0) is a generic instrument for assessing health and disability across different cultures and settings. WHODAS 2.0 generates standardized disability levels and profiles in all adult populations and across all diseases. This tool assesses 6 domains of functioning, including cognition, mobility, self-care, getting along, life activities, and participation. It is especially useful for grading the clinical effectiveness of rehabilitation interventions and for assessing health status and disability levels.[13]

The Global Burden of Diseases, Injuries, and Risk Factors Study 2017 (GBD 2017) methodology comprehensively assesses prevalence, incidence, and years lived with disability (YLDs) for 354 causes in 195 countries and territories, and at the subnational level for a subset of countries, from 1990 to 2017.[10,14] GBD 2017 is the most comprehensive worldwide observational epidemiologic study to date and describes mortality and morbidity from major diseases, injuries, and risk factors to health at global, national, and regional levels, allowing geographic comparisons of the effects of different diseases. Epidemiologic disability measures include YLDs as well as years of life lost

(YLLs) and disability-adjusted life years (DALYs). GBD 2017 datasets and other GBD resources and tools may be queried.[15]

DEMOGRAPHICS OF DISABILITY

Global disability trends indicated by GBD 2017[16] show that the total burden of disability increased by 52% between 1990 and 2017, the burden of disability is driven mainly by noncommunicable diseases, and disability from metabolic conditions such as type 2 diabetes and fatty liver disease is increased around the world and across all levels of development. In general, female individuals have had and continue to experience higher levels of disability than male individuals. YLDs may be indexed by sociodemographic index (SDI) grouping reflecting global income, education, and fertility development status.

GBD 2017 findings show that low back pain, headache disorders, and depressive disorders were the leading causes of disability globally in 2017 (as reflected by YLDs), and have been for almost 3 decades. Collectively, these 3 conditions caused nearly 1 in 5 YLDs worldwide in 2017. The number of all-age YLDs attributed to low back pain increased by 30.0% (27.9%–31.9%) from 1990 to 2017.[10] GBD 2017 reports disability-related datasets including "Incidence, Prevalence, and Years Lived with Disability 1990 to 2017," "Disability-Adjusted Life Years and Healthy Life Expectancy 1990 to 2017," and "Burden by Risk 1990 to 2017."[15]

GBD Country Profiles show what health problems cause the most deaths, the most premature deaths, and the most disability, as well as what risk factors drive the most death and disability combined in a given country, such as Nepal (http://www.healthdata.org/Nepal). Further, the GBD Compare visualization tool application for Nepal (http://ihmeuw.org/4nqp) allows comparison of health causes and risks and exploration of patterns and trends by age and gender.

Besides increasing global noncommunicable disease, the global population is aging, which compounds global disability burden given the increasing prevalence of disability in older individuals. Increasing disability prevalence with age reflects an accumulation of health risks, including chronic illness and injuries. Increased disability prevalence in the aged is relatively higher in developing countries than in developed countries and higher among women than men. Persons with a certain group of disorders, such as Down syndrome and post-polio syndrome, are prone to show signs of premature aging, such as decreased strength, gait dysfunction, deconditioning, presbycusis, and osteoporosis.[17] Also, they are more vulnerable to age-related conditions. The incidence of Alzheimer disease is higher in patients with Down syndrome, for example, and dementia in general is more prevalent in persons with intellectual dysfunction unrelated to Down syndrome.[17]

Global estimates of childhood disability rates vary considerably given different definitions and assessment tools used. Variation is most significant across low-income countries because of the lack of language-specific and culturally appropriate assessment tools that challenge identification and characterization of disabilities.[18] A literature review of low and middle-income countries reported disability prevalence of pediatric populations ranging from 0.4% to 12.7%.[19] The United Nations Children's Fund estimation of the number of children with disabilities was 150 million in 2005.[20]

The concept that disability is a product of the interaction between the individual and the environment is valid in children as in adults. A child's functioning should be viewed in the context of the family and social environment. Malnutrition, poor health, impoverishment, and an environment devoid of stimulus and motivation can all impair normal development and predispose the child to disability. A positive screen for risk of disability in a child revealed a positive correlation with growing up in poorer households; discrimination and restricted access to social services, including early-childhood education; underweight status and stunted growth; and severe parental physical punishment.

DISABILITY AND ENVIRONMENT

The ICF defines "environmental factors" in the context of health as "the physical, social, and attitudinal environment in which people live and conduct their lives." These factors can inhibit or facilitate a person's functioning. The effect of environmental factors on disability is complicated and often difficult to determine, as often multiple environmental risk factors for disability coexist and interact. The physical, social, and political aspects of environment require full consideration when evaluating an individual's health. Varied environmental conditions, such as poverty, poor sanitation, malnutrition, and lack of access to health care, are linked to increased disability. Disability (and mortality) incidence peaks during environmental emergencies, such as natural disasters or human conflict. The male life expectancy in Syria decreased by 11.3 years between 2005 and 2015[21] due to protracted civil war and its sequelae, for example. By contrast, facilitative environmental changes, such as improved access to transportation and public infrastructure, adaptive modifications to home or workplace, use of assistive devices and technologies, and campaigns to promote positive attitudes toward persons with disabilities (PWDs), lower disability prevalence by reducing environmental barriers. The person with a disability benefits from a positive interaction with the environment that promotes the achievement of health and life goals.[22]

DISABILITY, HUMAN RIGHTS, AND SOCIOECONOMIC INEQUALITY

The CRPD and other international documents have helped establish disability as a human rights issue. The CRPD delineates the social, cultural, civil, political, and economic rights of PWDs. It also outlines the principles of respect for inherent dignity, individual autonomy, nondiscrimination, participation and inclusion in society, respect for difference, equality of opportunity, accessibility, and respect for evolving capacities of children with disabilities.[23] PWDs are more likely to experience disrespect, prejudice, abuse, and frank violence than the general population. They are more often denied equal access to education, employment, or health care. Political participation and autonomy are more commonly denied in PWDs.[6,24] Human rights considerations factor significantly in the socioeconomics of disability as equitable health outcomes may be infeasible due to reduced access to health care resources from economic inequality. Moreover, PWDs have comparatively high health care costs because of the often chronic nature of their diseases and higher degree of comorbidities.

In most high-income countries, PWDs have disadvantaged access to education and employment. Accordingly, poverty rates in the working-age group are higher in PWDs than in the general population. Ireland, Australia, and Korea are among the countries in which poverty rates are highest; Sweden, Norway, Netherlands, Iceland, Slovakia, and Mexico are countries where rates are among the lowest.[25] A British longitudinal study suggested that employment rates fell with the onset of disability and continued to trend down with the duration of disability.[26] Most studies on the socioeconomic status of people with and without disabilities report cross-sectional data.

Research on the socioeconomic status of PWDs in developing countries is scarce but growing. The trend of worse educational and vocational outcomes in PWDs in developed countries is repeated in developing countries. Lower school attendance rates are found among children with disabilities in most cross-sectional studies on educational consumption.[27,28] A study of 15 developing countries suggests that health care expenditures are higher in households with disabled members than in those without disabled members.[29]

SUMMARY

Scientifically robust disability epidemiology at the global and national levels generates statistics on disability-related demographics, trends, and relationships between health-related variables. These data inform development of valid comparisons, accurate estimates, and targets for health improvement, which are increasingly used by disability and rehabilitation stakeholders to develop policies, programs, and services for persons in developing countries who experience disability. These essential rehabilitation interventions that demonstrate applied disaster epidemiology are helping to meet the profound global unmet need for rehabilitation,[8] fulfilling the necessary role of rehabilitation in achieving United Nations Sustainable Development Goal 3 to "ensure healthy lives and promote well-being for all at all ages."[30,31] Ongoing advance in disability epidemiology method, practice, and application is required to achieve desired levels of rehabilitation globally and especially in developing countries. Rehabilitation practitioners, including physiatrists, in these low-resource settings should be well aware of prevailing disability epidemiology dynamics to best serve their patients.

REFERENCES

1. United Nations Department of Economic and Social Affairs. Preamble to the convention on the right of persons with disabilities. Available at: https://www.un.org/development/desa/disabilities/convention-on-the-rights-of-persons-with-disabilities/preamble.html. Accessed December 21, 2018.
2. Wade DT. Epidemiology of disabling neurological disease: how and why does disability occur? J Neurol Neurosurg Psychiatry 1997;63(Suppl 1):S11–8.
3. Kostanjsek N. Use of The International Classification of Functioning, Disability and Health (ICF) as a conceptual framework and common language for disability statistics and health information systems. BMC Public Health 2011;11(Suppl 4):S3.
4. ICD 11. Available at: http://www.who.int/classifications/icd/en/. Accessed December 21, 2018.
5. World Health Organization. How to use the ICF: a practical manual for using the International Classification of Functioning, Disability and Health (ICF). Exposure draft for comment. Geneva (Switzerland): WHO; 2013.
6. World Health Organization, World Bank. World report on disability. Geneva (Switzerland): World Health Organization; 2011.
7. Drum CE, Krahn GL, Peterson JJ, et al. Health of people with disabilities: determinants and disparities. In: Drum CE, Krahn GL, Bersani H, editors. Disability and public health. 1st edition. Washington, DC: American Public Health Association; 2009. p. 125–44.
8. Rimmer JH, Rowland JL. Health promotion for people with disabilities: implications for empowering the person and promoting disability-friendly environments. J Lifestyle Med 2008;2:409–20.
9. Merikangas KR, Ames M, Cui L, et al. The impact of comorbidity of mental and physical conditions on role disability in the US adult household population. Arch Gen Psychiatry 2007;64(10):1180–8.

10. GBD 2017 Risk Factor Collaborators. Global, regional, and national comparative risk assessment of 84 behavioural, environmental and occupational, and metabolic risks or clusters of risks for 195 countries and territories, 1990-2017: a systematic analysis for the Global Burden of Disease Study 2017. Lancet 2018; 392(10159):1923–94.

11. Kamenov K, Mills JA, Chatterji S, et al. Needs and unmet needs for rehabilitation services: a scoping review. Disabil Rehabil 2019;41(10):1227–37.

12. World Health Organization. Rehabilitation 2030 a call for action: health information systems and rehabilitation. Meeting report. Geneva, (Switzerland); World Health Organization; 2017. Available: https://www.who.int/rehabilitation/rehab-2030-call-for-action/en/. Accessed December 21, 2018.

13. World Health Organization. WHO disability assessment Schedule 2.0 (WHODAS 2.0). 2018. Available at: https://www.who.int/classifications/icf/whodasii/en/. Accessed December 21, 2018.

14. Global burden of disease (GBD). 2018. Available at: http://www.healthdata.org/gbd. Accessed December 21, 2018.

15. Global burden of disease study 2017 (GBD 2017) data resources. 2018. Available at: http://ghdx.healthdata.org/gbd-2017. Accessed December 21, 2018.

16. Institute for Health Metrics and Evaluation. Global trends in disability. Available at: http://www.healthdata.org/sites/default/files/files/infographics/Infographic_GBD2017-YLDs-Highlights_2018.pdf. Accessed December 21, 2018.

17. Australian Institute of Health and Welfare (AIHW). Disability and ageing: Australian population patterns and implications. Canberra (Australia): Australian Institute of Health and Welfare; 2000.

18. Hartley S, Newton CRJC. Children with developmental disabilities in the majority of the world. In: Shevell M, editor. Neurodevelopmental disabilities: clinical and scientific foundations. 1st edition. London: Mac Keith Press for the International Child Neurology Association; 2009. p. 70–84.

19. Maulik PK, Darmstadt GL. Childhood disability in low- and middle-income countries: overview of screening, prevention, services, legislation, and epidemiology. Pediatrics 2007;120(Suppl 1):S1–55.

20. The state of the world's children 2006: excluded and invisible. New York: The United Nations Children's Fund; 2005. Available: https://www.unicef.org/publications/index_30398.html. Accessed December 21, 2018.

21. The Lancet. GBD 2015: from big data to meaningful change. Lancet 2016; 388(10053):1447.

22. Stiens SA, Shamberg S, Shamberg A, et al. Environmental barriers: solutions for participation, collaboration, and togetherness. In: O'Young BJ, Young MA, Stiens SA, editors. Physical medicine and rehabilitation secrets. 3rd edition. Philadelphia: Mosby; 2007. p. 76–85.

23. United Nations Department of Economic and Social Affairs. Convention on the Rights of Persons with Disabilities. Available at: https://www.un.org/development/desa/disabilities/convention-on-the-rights-of-persons-with-disabilities.html. Accessed December 21, 2018.

24. Quinn G, Degener T. A survey of international, comparative and regional disability law reform. In: Breslin ML, Yee S, editors. Disability rights law and policy: international and national perspectives. 1st edition. Leiden (Netherlands): Brill - Nijhoff; 2002. p. 3–129.

25. Organisation for Economic Co-operation and Development Directorate for Employment, Labour and Social Affairs. Sickness, disability and work: keeping

on track in the economic downturn. Paris: Organisation for Economic Co-operation and Development; 2009.

26. Jenkins SP, Rigg JA. Disability and disadvantage: selection, onset, and duration effects 2003. Available at: https://core.ac.uk/download/pdf/93877.pdf.

27. Eide AH, van Rooy G, Loeb ME. Living conditions among people with activity limitations in Namibia: a representative, national study. SINTEF report. 2003.

28. Eide AH, Loeb ME. Living conditions among people with activity limitations in Zambia. A national representative study. 2006. Available at: http://www.safod.net/library/files/m53808.pdf.

29. Mitra S, Posarac A, Vick B. Disability and poverty in developing countries: a snapshot from the world health survey. Washington, DC: Human Development Network Social Protection; 2011.

30. Rehabilitation 2030: a call for action. Available at: http://www.who.int/rehabilitation/rehab-2030/en/. Accessed December 21, 2018.

31. Gimigliano F, Negrini S. The World Health Organization "Rehabilitation 2030: a call for action". Eur J Phys Rehabil Med 2017;53(2):155–68.

Concept Changes and Standardizing Tools in Community-Based Rehabilitation

Wouter De Groote, MD, PRM

KEYWORDS

- Community-based rehabilitation • Community-based inclusive development
- Primary health care • Capacity building • Standards

KEY POINTS

- Community-based rehabilitation is changing from basic service delivery in rehabilitation to a rights-based approach holding local authorities accountable for inclusive measures in all aspects of life.
- For low- and middle-income countries, medical rehabilitation at the community level needs to be defined regarding its workforce, relation to primary health care, and institutionalized rehabilitation.
- Meanwhile, the evidence base for community-based rehabilitation is growing as a guide for implementation. A process of standardization to scale up is proposed.

INTRODUCTION

Community-based rehabilitation (CBR) was introduced by the World Health Organization (WHO) in 1976.

The primary concept of CBR at that time was that rehabilitation should be home based, given to the person with a disability, with their family and caregivers supported by local community members who were typically health workers. CBR programs focused primarily on bringing practical rehabilitation techniques to the community level when these skills were unavailable at hospitals or health centers in low- and middle-income countries.

Over the next 3 to 4 decades, CBR has changed considerably at the level of concepts and practice, mostly influenced by the development sector. The Twin Track approach was introduced in CBR practice, enabling an individual with independent living skills (through service provision) and addressing equalization of opportunities resulting in inclusion (through advocacy).

Disclosure Statement: The author has nothing to disclose.
Rehabilitation Department, AZ Rivierenland, Kasteelstraat 23, Bornem 2880, Belgium
E-mail address: Wouter.de.groote@telenet.be

1047-9651/19/© 2019 Elsevier Inc. All rights reserved.

In 2004, the Joint Position Paper issued by the International Labour Organization (ILO), United Nations Educational, Scientific and Cultural Organization (UNESCO), and WHO defined CBR as "a general strategy within community development for the rehabilitation, poverty reduction, equalization of opportunities and social inclusion of all people with disabilities."[1]

COMMUNITY-BASED REHABILITATION AND REHABILITATION

The same Joint Position Paper describes CBR as having a multisectoral approach, which operates at a community level to promote people with disabilities accessing services available to all other community members and focuses on their social, community, and economic inclusion.

Although rehabilitation techniques remain a component of CBR, one now addresses 5 key pillars: health, education, livelihood, social, and empowerment.[2] The multisectoral approach is represented in the 5 components of the WHO CBR matrix (**Fig. 1**). CBR programs work for the benefit and development of the whole community, encouraging inclusive development, postering empowerment, and emphasizing the realization for human rights for all.[3] As such, CBR is the strategy to achieve community-based inclusive development (CBID). The CBR strategy can set up an ideal framework to implement the provisions of the UN Convention on the Rights of Persons with a Disability.[1]

Until now, the term "CBR" has stood the test of time, but in 2011, Maya Thomas[4] mentions the remaining interest groups in the disability sector who object to the term "CBR" on the grounds that including the word "rehabilitation" makes it medical as opposed to rights based, and therefore, not "politically correct."

Today, it seems that the name of CBR is actually being changed into a name that reflects the rights-based approach. With the name change comes a definition change as well: "Community Based Inclusive Development is a rights-based approach within community development for the equalization of opportunities, empowerment and social inclusion of all people with disabilities."[5] CBID builds further on the momentum of the UN Convention for the Rights of People with a Disability, which emphasizes "the

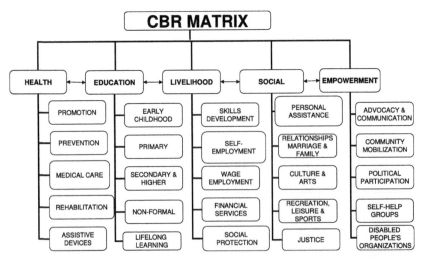

Fig. 1. WHO CBR matrix. (*From* World Health Organization. CBR matrix. Available at: https://www.who.int/disabilities/cbr/cbr_matrix_11.10.pdf; with permission.)

importance of mainstreaming disability issues as an integral part of relevant strategies of sustainable development" (UNCRPD [UN Convention on the Rights of Persons with Disabilities], preamble g, 2007). CBID aims at supporting people with disabilities, their family, and organizations, ensuring equal participation in their community and equal access to services.

At this point, health-related rehabilitation is no longer part of the definition. Rehabilitation at a community level is no longer a component as such and has become a service like any other. The goal of CBID is to improve access to services, not to deliver services. The key words of CBID are capacity building, community mobilization, peer support, Disabled People's Organization, and nondiscrimination, which are all elements in the "social" and "empowerment" components of the former WHO CBR matrix (see **Fig. 1**).

When looking at the shift made over the past 4 decades, CBR was addressing basic rehabilitation techniques to an individual with a disability to develop independent living skills at first, whereas CBID's interventions aim for inclusive policies and inclusive service delivery. The WHO CBR Matrix is reduced to its social and empowerment pillars. Service delivery in rehabilitation as an integral part of the intervention's scope has been left out, whereas interventions now work toward empowerment. People with disabilities should be able to exercise their rights by giving them the tools and peer support, while local government or other duty bearers are held accountable.

Together with this name and definition change, a disappearance of an indirect link with people with a disability is also noted because CBID is a general concept that applies for every minority group (**Box 1**).

For the believers of CBR, it is argued that conceptually, there is a need for more clarity about the positioning of CBID related to CBR. Will CBR remain an integral part of CBID, because it is the strategy to achieve the goal of CBID, meaning that the UNCRPD is the overarching principle of CBR? Or will the opposite happen, with CBID becoming an integral part of CBR? According to current findings, CBID is addressing 2 out of 5 CBR components. In this case, the rights-based approach could become the driving force for CBR. Or is CBR actually being replaced by a name and concept that better reflects the rights-based approach? In these matters, Maya Thomas already warned us about confusion among field-level practitioners and, in the long run, a danger of diluting the only approach that is still seen as the most appropriate one for developing countries.[3]

In a rights-based model, mainly consisting of capacity building, advocacy, and sensitization activities, people with a disability will ask for their right to receive individualized medical rehabilitation! In the area of health, CBR was able to make a particular contribution in providing these health services as close as possible to people's own communities, including in rural areas (UNCRPD, article 25c).

In low- and middle-income countries, at this point, primary care level service delivery mainly aims at providing services in the promotion, prevention, and treatment of health conditions. Although CBID wants to provide a person with a disability with the necessary tools to advocate for inclusive rehabilitation, it is appealing for

Box 1
Conceptual change of community-based rehabilitation to community-based inclusive development

CBR (1976):	Individualized	Rehabilitation	Single sector	Service delivery	Disability	WHO
CBID (2019):	Mainstreaming	Inclusion	Multisectoral	Advocacy	Minority group	UN agencies

autonomy and responsibility of the group of persons with a disability, in the context of local authorities with reduced implementing power and poorly available rehabilitation services. A similar concern is shared by the CBR Africa Network pointing out that the continent is not ready for a conceptual change. Still much work must be done in terms of leveling the ground necessary for the change to be effective, mostly with regards to inherent negative attitudes in the community and among government stakeholders.[6]

WHAT ABOUT "REHABILITATION"?

Although CBID is being promoted among different UN agencies, there is a strong momentum going on for rehabilitation at WHO: "Rehabilitation 2030: A Call for Action" asks for coordinated and concerted action to scale up rehabilitation services and address the profound unmet needs by integrating rehabilitation in national health strategic planning, at all layers (tertiary to primary and community level). When moving toward integrated person-centered care especially, it is imperative that quality rehabilitation is embedded in service delivery models.[7]

The WHO describes rehabilitation as "a set of interventions designed to optimize functioning and reduce disability in individuals with health conditions in interaction with their environment." It is important to know that "rehabilitation may be needed by anyone with a health condition who experiences some form of limitation in functioning," which means that the target group for rehabilitation becomes much larger than the group of "persons with disabilities."

The good thing is that WHO now stands for rehabilitation at a community level, among others, as an integrated part of the mainstream health care system, whereas it is advocating for ministries of health to take up a responsible role. However, it is still unclear what community-delivered rehabilitation will look like, and how it will relate to the primary health care level, or even merge with it. Community-delivered rehabilitation at least should be integrated within the health care system, complementing institution-based services. For the strengthening of rehabilitation in low-resources countries, there is no time to lose, because the recent changes are leaving an important gap behind. In 1993, Helander stated that CBR was initiated in the early 1980s because of a failure of the conventional system of rehabilitation then prevalent in many developing countries. Today, (increasing) unmet needs are still being faced. When CBID does not focus on rehabilitation service delivery as a core intervention, community-delivered rehabilitation needs to come from a top-down approach by the Ministry of Health. Meanwhile, the major problem of outpatient institution-based rehabilitation in low-resource settings remains unchanged. It is a set of interventions that often needs to be repeated frequently; although the people that are in need of rehabilitation usually have transport issues, they are not able to access services that are centralized. In Malawi, the uptake of referral services for children with a disability has been demonstrated to be very low with transport difficulties, lack of information, and financial constraints being the most common reasons for nonuptake.[8] For rehabilitation services in the late postacute setting and in chronic conditions, it does not make sense to organize it in a centralized manner. There seems to be only 1 solution: bring services closer to homes. Of course, some rehabilitation services can only be organized at a central level (eg, mobility aids provision), but very frequent visits to a rehabilitation center at least should be avoided to reduce out-of-pocket expenditure for transport in a population that is generally poor.

The takeaway message for community health workers as concluded from the 73rd UN General Assembly about noncommunicable diseases also accounts for community rehabilitation workers: "improved training and education are needed, and there is an opportunity to re-design health systems to revolutionize health care." For low-resource settings or any country with access issues related to transport, a new cadre in the rehabilitation workforce will need to be conceived, which delivers basic rehabilitation skills at home. This new cadre needs to be defined as per its relation to the other members of the rehabilitation team that are institutionalized. The main characteristic of the community rehabilitation worker's intervention will be the sharing of information and basic techniques that are safe to be executed by the client or caregiver, without the supervision of an expert. These interventions mostly relate to the International Classification of Functioning, Disability, and Health (ICF) components of participation, environment, and personal factors (**Box 2**).

FINDING CONSENSUS IN COMMUNITY-BASED REHABILITATION

Meanwhile, CBR continues to evolve,[6] and the current conceptual debate does not stop the call for strengthening the evidence base for CBR as a guide for implementation. A certain challenge is being presented here as, with the development of the CBR guidelines, it is understood that a single model for CBR does not exist. Building evidence is challenging when an important variety is the rule. CBR nowadays is too diverse to market and still too undefined to rely on in an overall strategic plan. Whenever a CBR program is (partially) state funded, it is probably a local service provider using state money for community activities. Rarely, CBR activities result from national strategic planning. A lack of awareness and recognition of proven added value at the level of policymakers are being faced owing to an absence of consistency. Nevertheless, as an answer to public health issues related to disability and the diversity of needs expressed by a person with a disability, many people are still believers of the CBR strategy.

Building evidence could begin with basic multistakeholder consensus as a start for implementation research. When the CBR guidelines provide an overview of all possible intervention areas, which may be used with a "pick-and-mix" approach, there is a need to find consensus about the minimal standards that involve content, implementation methodology, human resources, training curricula, support system, and so forth. To scale up means to set a reproducible standard, which, in the case of CBR, should perfectly be able to provide an answer to the gap identified by a needs-based approach for a person with a disability in his or her living environment. A standardization process would facilitate the development of international standards

---

Box 2
Relationship institution-based rehabilitation and community-delivered rehabilitation

	Institution-Based Rehabilitation	Community-Delivered Rehabilitation
ICF components	Body function and structure, activity	Participation, environment, personal factors
Pathway	Acute and postacute setting	Chronic conditions
Guidance	Expert supervision	Autorehabilitation
Therapy type	Passive and active therapy	Active therapy
Therapy frequency	Repetition	Single context-based intervention
Mean	Applied technology	Transfer of knowledge
Timeframe	Time-bound intervention	Continuous monitoring
Infrastructure	Equipment	Home setting
Work out	Diagnosis and treatment	Detection and referral
Competencies	Technical support	Task shifting

and recognition of CBR professionals, because it will enable policymakers to position CBR activities within their strategic planning.

An example is the CBR field worker as the core human resource. At the CBR Global Network conference in Kuala Lumpur in 2016, it was concluded that "we are still facing a lack of recognition of the CBR field worker, left without accountability and certificates, mainly due to a variety of duties…" Indeed, recognition of the CBR field worker depends on a clear job description and well-defined training curriculum. Nowadays, training programs are all different in terms of their content and duration and offered by a variety of providers. For example, in some countries, tertiary institutions offer a diploma course for CBR personnel, whereas, in other countries, training programs may not be accredited and may only last for a few weeks or months.[2] As a result of this diversity in training approaches and different inputs of CBR program planners, CBR programs also differ at the level of content, quality, and methodology.

The global CBR community therefore should promote research about the standards of the CBR building blocks and facilitate its systematic application and evaluation.

THE PROCESS OF STANDARDIZING

Finkenflügel and colleagues[3] mention that many classification models for CBR have been developed to create conceptual order, but none of the models appears to be widely accepted (**Box 3**). They have found 16 documents describing 11 different models. None of the classification models directs strongly to a certain type of program that is seen as superior to the others. All models are framing realities and not advocating a specific type of "rehabilitation in the community."

Box 3
Standardization of building blocks in community-based rehabilitation

Building Block	Standardizing Document
Concept	CBR guidelines and WHO CBR Matrix, INCLUDE
M&E	3 Domains (Wirz and Thomas, 2002)
	Monitoring Manual and Menu (University of Sydney, 2014)
	CBR Indicators Manual (WHO, 2015)
	Participatory Inclusion Evaluation or PIE (Post et al, 2016)
HR skills	Toward a core set of clinical skills for Health-Related CBR (O'Dowd et al, 2015)
	Recommendations for Guidelines for the Rehabilitation Workforce (MacLachlan et al, 2013)
	Development of essential standards for field worker training in disability inclusion (CBR/CBID)
HR entry profile	Development of essential standards for field worker training in disability inclusion (CBR/CBID)
Supportive environment	Development of essential standards for field worker training in disability inclusion (CBR/CBID)
Training	CBR matrix and perceived training needs of CBR workers (Deepak et al, 2011)
	Recommendations for Guidelines for the Rehabilitation Workforce (MacLachlan et al, 2013)
	Development of essential standards for field worker training in disability inclusion (CBR/CBID)
Financing	?
Management tools	?
Information system	?
M&E, Monitoring and Evaluation; HR, Human Resources	

The CBR Guidelines by WHO, ILO, UNESCO, and International Disability and Development Consortium in 2010 served as the first step to provide a unified understanding of the *concepts* and principles of CBR.[9] The core of these guidelines is the WHO CBR matrix, reflecting the multisectoral approach and providing a structure for CBR planners and practitioners. The guidelines suggest possible goals, desirable outcomes and activities for the different elements, and components of the matrix. It also provides guidance for program management: generally accepted tools that are used in program cycle management are applied to the CBR context. These tools include Strengths, Weaknesses, Opportunities and Threads (SWOT) analysis, problem tree, logical framework, Specific Measurable Realistic Acceptable and Timebound (SMART) principle for indicators, Gantt Chart, and Data collection methods. However, setting a conceptual standard, the CBR guidelines are lacking specified applications because no tools were specifically developed for CBR. Also, the guidelines are not prescriptive and may be used with a "pick-and-mix" approach.

Based on the CBR guidelines, an online program was established in 2016. Guiding users through different information modules, INCLUDE aims to support and inform CBR managers and interested stakeholders. A unified understanding of CBR implementation is the result.[10]

Looking at the systematic outcome and impact *evaluation*, Wirz and Thomas[11] provided a systematic evaluation framework focusing on 3 domains: maximizing the potential of a person with a disability, service delivery, and the environment. They have demonstrated that many indicators are being used and that grouping them is a valuable exercise in order to move beyond evaluations that are merely descriptions of activities.

Finkenflügel and colleagues[12] found 17 articles on the evaluation of projects. They show that programs develop program-specific evaluation instruments that might very well address the needs of the people involved in that project but make a comparison between programs and arduous exercise.

In April 2014, the "Monitoring Manual and Menu (MM&M) for CBR and other community-based disability inclusive development programs" provided a comprehensive overview of the monitoring of CBR programs, looking at preparation, information design, monitoring plan, and review.[13] This manual was conceived for 2 main reasons: (1) to build evidence about the efficacy of CBR; (2) to create internal and external consistency among the variety of monitoring tools for CBR programs, respectively, between the stages of the monitoring plan and across the studies.

Then, the CBR indicators manual appeared containing quantitative indicators capable of capturing the difference CBR makes in the lives of people with disabilities, between adults, youth, and children, and those without disabilities, in the areas of health, education, social life, livelihood, and empowerment.[14] As the WHO CBR matrix is used as the theoretic framework, the CBR indicators manual is considered a comprehensive evaluation instrument, not being program specific and still enabling comparison.

Because CBR/CBID is thriving for inclusive development and the CBR indicators manual does not include persons with a disability in the decision-making process, there was a need for another evaluation tool measuring impact in CBR. Participatory inclusion evaluation (PIE) is a flexible approach developed as an answer to the need for a more structured approach to impact evaluations of CBR programs that are inclusive and participatory. PIE is conceptualized in an evaluation framework, using both quantitative and qualitative evaluation methods. It involves the participation of 3 types of stakeholders: people with disabilities, the CBR core team, and the network of strategic partners. The impact is defined as changes in inclusion, empowerment, and living conditions. Summarizing findings and reporting are still promoted to be linked with the

CBR matrix.[15] The use of PIE is supported by an expert panel that reached consensus on key features of best evaluative practices in CBR.[16]

At the level of *human resources*, Deepak and colleagues[17] describe the most pressing perceived learning needs for the different domains of the CBR matrix, and for different kinds of disabilities. They selected the 3 most important overall learning needs per CBR worker. This exercise resulted in a list of 14 topics. According to the CBR workers, the most common learning needs are those related to the area of empowerment mostly, and livelihood and health (medical rehabilitation). This study gives us an interesting insight into the development of training programs. On the other hand, it is not clear whether the perceived training needs reflected the CBR program content or CBR field worker educational background. Many field workers have different profiles, which result in different training needs. In order to describe a standardized training curriculum, these confounding factors will need to be eliminated.

"Recommendations for Guidelines for the Rehabilitation Workforce: A Realist Synthesis" (2013) describes the interaction between the health sector and CBR, and thus, the community rehabilitation workforce. Research questions are designed to investigate competencies, training, capacity building, minimum requirements for service delivery, and so forth. It is mentioned here that health-related aspects of rehabilitation should not exist in isolation from broader aspects of the rights of people with disabilities. Except for health-related rehabilitation skills, the CBR worker is also required to have skills in at least some of the other areas of the CBR matrix.[18] Derived from a systemic literature review, the investigators could not identify specific clinical skills for health-related rehabilitation.

In 2015, O'Dowd and colleagues[19] describe a core set of work activities relating to the health component of CBR. Notably, they discovered that, still, 8 out of 10 most frequently used skills are of a generalized nature and less discipline specific (eg, referrals, advocacy, psychosocial support), independent of the educational background of the CBR worker. This finding demonstrates the need of a client in the community context. According to the investigators, it shows that CBR is mainly targeting the ICF components of "environment" and "personal factors." Nevertheless, a discrepancy between the skills used most frequently and those that are ranked as most important by the CBR worker is noted. This finding is specifically the case for home-based rehabilitation, which is consistently ranked as very important but does not appear in the top 10 list of the most frequently used skills.

Finally, the "Development of essential standards for field worker training in disability inclusion (CBR/CBID)" is a document to be submitted for publication. It uses empirical evidence for the identification of standards for the profile, training curriculum, and support system of a CBR/CBID field worker. Data are collected across many settings, which help to build consensus about minimal findings that are cross cutting. The investigators plead for a consensus and due respect to the CBR/CBID field workers, about their entry level recommendations, competency framework, and supportive environment.

INTRODUCTION OF AN INTERNATIONAL CLASSIFICATION OF FUNCTIONING, DISABILITY, AND HEALTH–BASED ASSESSMENT AND INTERVENTION MODEL IN COMMUNITY-BASED REHABILITATION

The author would like to contribute to the standardizing process in CBR with an assessment and intervention model. As a CBR program planner, the author considers CBR and its interventions to be a first entry or primary care level of support to a person with a disability. Based on the CBR Guidelines, a possible advantage of CBR is its holistic approach, looking at all aspects that need to be fulfilled to have a full partici-pative life. However, the danger of a comprehensive approach is that it is not applied completely, and especially not providing a tailor-made answer to the need of every person within the same zone of action, because a tremendous diversity of possible in-terventions might result in less appropriate measures at the individual level. In order to individualize a needs-based intervention, one should visit the home of every person to understand the complexity of the needs.

When a CBR field worker visits a new client at home, he or she has to be equipped with a standardized model of assessment. This assessment tool should consist of a comprehensive evaluation method covering the multifaceted needs of a person living with a disability in relation to the environment. In addition, within the same assess-ment, there should be a way to prioritize. Most CBR field workers say they are over-whelmed by the amount and diversity of needs. They often do not know the answer to all questions, and they do not know where to start. Defining a priority need therefore is crucial: it is an important step in case management that facilitates a successful outcome of the intervention.

In 2011, it has been demonstrated that the ICF is a relevant and potentially useful framework and classification, providing building blocks for the systematic recording of information in CBR monitoring and evaluation.[20] The ICF model fits the require-ments to serve as a framework for overall assessment in CBR because it describes well the different components that influence and compose a disability experience. As such, an ICF-based assessment model is proposed, which will enable the assessor to map all major issues within the different components of the ICF model (**Box 4**).

Box 4
International Classification of Functioning, Disability, and Health–based assessment for community-based rehabilitation

1. Body function and structure   VAS 1:

   - Describe functional deficits (sensory, motor, mental, mixed, and so forth):
   - Other functional issues (eg, incontinence, seizures, pain, contractures):

2. Activity   VAS 1:

   - Mobility at home (transfer, moving around):
   - Activities of daily living (ADL: dress, bath, eat, drink):
   - Household activities (cooking, gardening, cleaning, washing clothes):

3. Participation   VAS 1:

   - Mobility in community (transport, accessibility of infrastructure):
   - Education/professional activity:
   - Inclusion in the community (attitudes, discrimination, inclusive policies applied):
   - Sexuality:

4. Environment   VAS 1:

   - At home (accessibility, lack of home adaptations for ADL):
   - Caregivers and family (attitude, compliance, and burden of care):

5. Personal factors   VAS 1:

   - Psychology (emotions, depression, and isolation) of the client:
   - Compliance of the client toward proposed interventions:

In the "body function and structure" component, the CBR field worker wants to get an idea of a motor, sensory, mental, or mixed disability. There is no use of medical diagnosis at this level; a description of the type of disability is sufficient. He or she might also evaluate any related problem or comorbidity (eg, communication, joint

---

Box 5
International Classification of Functioning, Disability, and Health–based interventions for community-based rehabilitation

Body function and structure
- Provision of home-based rehabilitation (M)
- Referral to medical rehabilitation service provider (M)
- Referral to medical service provider (M)
- Encourage person with disability to have health insurance (M)

Activity
- Referral for assistive devices (mobility and other) (M)
- Home-based rehabilitation about activities of daily living (M)
- Encourage family life participation (S)

Participation
- Collaborate with health service providers to make services accessible (M)
- Advise on mobility in the community and lobby for community facilities to be accessible (S)
- Raise community awareness about UNCRPD and stigmatization (S)
- Education: awareness raising at school, enroll and support children in school, school adaptations, motivate family to support children's education, advocate and build capacity of selected schools on inclusive education, home-based learning (Ed)
- Professional integration: referral to Direct Support Programs, facilitate vocational skills training, support to start up business and microcredit, assist trained persons to seek jobs, and advocate with employers to give opportunity for persons with disabilities (L)
- Referral to Social Protection Programs, encourage persons with disabilities to participate in cultural activity, organize inclusive sports and games (S)
- Support persons with disabilities and families to access legal assistance and justice (S)
- Encourage persons with disabilities to participate in the national election process (Em)
- Lobby for inclusive policies at local authorities (Em)
- Education about sexuality (M)

Environment
- Home adaptations (M)
- Training of family members on how to take care of persons with disabilities (M, Em)
- Behavioral change training for caregiver (M)

Personal factors
- Communication skills training (support materials for communication) (Em)
- Establish and train CBR Committees and self-help groups (Em)
- Encourage disabled people organization membership (Em)
- Psychosocial counseling to person with a disability (M, S)

WHO CBR matrix pillars: Ed, education; Em, empowerment; L, livelihood; M, medical; S, social.

stiffness, spasticity, paralysis, incontinence, epilepsy). Then, the component of "activity" is assessed with questions about mobility at home, activities of daily living, and household activities. For the "participation" component, it is suggested to ask about mobility in the community, educational and professional activities, inclusion in the community, and sexuality. The "environment" component is checked with home accessibility and adaptations, and the attitude of caregivers. Finally, for "personal factors," one evaluates psychological characteristics and the compliance of the client.

At this point, CBR field workers will have an overview of the disability experience consisting of a brief description of every ICF component. The next step is to get an idea of how these components relatively define the disability experience, evaluating the perceived burden for every ICF component separately, and to turn this evaluation into an expressed need, with a possibility to prioritize. A reversed visual analogue scale (VAS) with culturally neutral faces has been field tested several times by CBR International for these purposes. It is introduced to the person with a disability or caregiver right after the assessment of every ICF component.

Oppositely, a numeric score of 10 is used to have an idea of the subjective importance of this component. Zero corresponds with a very sad face, meaning that this aspect has a high negative impact on the person's life. A 10 corresponds with a smiling face, meaning that the client has no worries about it. As a result, the CBR field worker will have 5 scores on 10 (1 score for every ICF component) with the lowest score for the component with the most negative impact on the person's life. This component represents the prioritized need for which intervention should be suggested. Of course, the person with disabilities or caregiver should first be confronted with the findings, and the outcome is still open for discussion. In case of a tie especially, there should be a conversation about how to prioritize further. As such, the person with a disability will be able to express their most important problem, and the assessor will be able to get a comprehensive idea of the person's experience on his or her disabilities and still focus on 1 item at a time.

Once the person with a disability agrees with the outlined priority need, the CBR field worker will propose an intervention that answers to the need and fits within the same ICF component. In almost every case, the intervention will have a link with the WHO CBR matrix (**Box 5**). The intervention should have a starting and an ending date, which needs to be agreed on mutually by both the user and the CBR field worker. At the end of the intervention, the reversed VAS is again presented to the person with a disability to score the outcome of the intervention. An increase of 2 points is considered a success, and another intervention may then be proposed. In case of no success, it is possible to set another ending date for the same intervention when it is concluded that it is still realistic to improve in these matters.

SUMMARY

CBR has considerably changed in the past 4 decades, resulting in a rights-based approach holding local authorities responsible for service delivery. For medical rehabilitation, there is a concern about how this gap will be covered. Meanwhile, the CBR community is still asking to strengthen the evidence base for CBR implementation, recognizing its extensiveness and variety on the ground. The creation of standardizing tools will favor this process because it provides the building blocks to scale up and sets a standard for implementation research. Finally, an ICF-based assessment and intervention model for CBR is proposed.

REFERENCES

1. ILO, UNESCO, WHO. CBR: a strategy for rehabilitation, equalization of opportunities, poverty reduction and social inclusion of people with disabilities. joint position paper 2004. New York.
2. Faculty of Health Sciences, University of Sydney, Australia. Review of diploma of community based rehabilitation at Solomon Islands. Sydney (Australia): National University; 2015. Available at: http://sydney.edu.au/health-sciences/whocc-rehabilitation/. Accessed June 24, 2018.
3. Finkenflügel H, Cornielje H, Velema J. The use of classification models in the evaluation of CBR programmes. Disabil Rehabil 2008;30(5):348–54.
4. Thomas M. Reflections on community-based rehabilitation. Psychol Dev Soc J 2011;23(2):277–91.
5. International Disability and Development Consortium. Briefing paper: community-based inclusive development (CBID) 2018. Brussels (Belgium).
6. CBR Africa Network. AfriCAN Newsletter. 2018. Available at: https://gallery.mailchimp.com/458c63b4dc1f273ceb29346aa/files/01cd8abb-7d8c-4809-9c41-a43852a16300/2018_newsletter.pdf. Accessed February 3, 2019.
7. WHO. Rehabilitation 2030: a call for action. rehabilitation, key for health in de 21ste century. Geneva, 2017. Available at: https://www.who.int/rehabilitation/rehab-2030/en/. Accessed December 12, 2018.
8. London School of Hygiene & Tropical Medicine. Uptake of health and rehabilitation referrals for children in Malawi, Findings from field research and in Malawi and current literature 2014. London. Available at: http://disabilitycentre.lshtm.ac.uk/files/2014/07/MalawiAccessSummaryReport.pdf. Accessed February 19, 2019.
9. WHO. CBR Guidelines by WHO, ILO, UNESCO and IDDC 2010. Geneva (Switzerland). Available at: https://www.who.int/disabilities/cbr/guidelines/en/. Accessed November 12, 2018.
10. WHO. Include: a community-based rehabilitation (CBR) learning community 2016. Geneva (Switzerland). Available at: http://include.edc.org/. Accessed November 12, 2018.
11. Wirz S, Thomas M. Evaluation of community-based rehabilitation programmes: a search for appropriate indicators. Int J Rehabil Res 2002;25(3):163–71.
12. Finkenflügel H, Wolffers I, Huijsman R. The evidence base for community-based rehabilitation: a literature review. Int J Rehabil Res 2005;28(3):187–201.
13. Center for Disability Research and Policy, University of Sydney. Monitoring Manual and Menu (MM&M) for CBR and other community-based disability inclusive development programs 2014. Sydney (Austalia). Available at: http://sydney.edu.au/health-sciences/cdrp/projects/cbr-monitoring.shtml. Accessed January 10, 2019.
14. WHO. Community-based rehabilitation indicators manual 2015. Geneva (Switzerland). Available at: https://www.who.int/disabilities/cbr/cbr_indicators_manual/en/. Accessed December 14, 2018.
15. Post E, Cornielje H, Andrae K, et al. Participatory inclusion evaluation: a flexible approach to building the evidence base on the impact of community-based rehabilitation and inclusive development programmes. Knowl Manag Dev J 2016;11(2):7–26.
16. Grandisson M, Thibeault R, Hébert M, et al. Expert consensus on best evaluative practices in community-based rehabilitation. Disabil Rehabil 2016;38(5):499–510.

17. Deepak S, Kumar J, Ortali F, et al. CBR matrix and perceived training needs of CBR workers: a multi-country study. Disability, CBR and Inclusive Development 2011;22(1):85–98.
18. MacLachlan M, Gilmore B, McClean C, et al. Recommendations for guidelines for the rehabilitation workforce: a realist synthesis. Human Resources for Health; 2013. p. 41–5.
19. O'Dowd J, MacLachlan M, Khasnabis C, et al. Towards a core set of clinical skills for health-related community-based rehabilitation in low and middle income countries. Disability, CBR and Inclusive Development 2015;26(3):5–43.
20. Madden RH, Dune T, Lukersmith S, et al. The relevance of the International Classification of Functioning, Disability and Health (ICF) in monitoring and evaluating community-based rehabilitation (CBR). Disabil Rehabil 2014;36(10):826–37.

Rehabilitation in Disaster Relief

Fary Khan, MBBS, MD, FAFRM (RACP)[a,b,c,d], Bhasker Amatya, DMedSc, MD, MPH[a,b,*],
Su Yi Lee, MBBS, FAFRM (RACP)[a,b], Vandana Vasudevan, MBBS, FAFRM (RACP)[a]

KEYWORDS

- Rehabilitation • Natural disaster • Disability • Trauma

KEY POINTS

- In natural disasters, there is a significant increase in survivors with complex and long-term disabling injuries, signifying the need for rehabilitation.
- Despite growing demand, skilled rehabilitation workforce and services are limited in many disaster-prone countries, highlighting the burden of rehabilitation for individuals (their families) and community.
- Evidence supports early involvement of rehabilitation programs to minimize mortality, decrease disability, and improve functional outcomes and participation for disaster survivors.
- Medical rehabilitation is integral to disaster management and should be initiated acutely during emergency response and in the continuum of care.
- World Health Organization guidelines for Emergency Medical Team deployment in disasters have been developed, but are yet to be empirically implemented or validated.

INTRODUCTION

Natural disasters (eg, earthquakes, storms, tropical cyclone, landslide, drought, floods) are escalating worldwide.[1] Concomitant, human exposure and/or impact on population and society from these disaster are intensifying, owing to factors such as climate change, population growth, urbanization, density within living area, mass population displacements, and poorly planned infrastructure.[2] Between 2000 and

Disclosure Statement: This work was supported by internal resources of the Department of Rehabilitation, Royal Melbourne Hospital, Australia.
[a] Department of Rehabilitation, Royal Melbourne Hospital, Australian Rehabilitation Research Centre, Building 21, Royal Park Campus, 34-54 Poplar Road, Parkville, Victoria 3052, Australia; [b] Department of Medicine, University of Melbourne, Parkville, Victoria, Australia; [c] School of Public Health and Preventative Medicine, Monash University, Clayton, Victoria, Australia; [d] Disability Inclusive Unit, Nossal Institute of Global Health, University of Melbourne, Parkville, Victoria, Australia
* Corresponding author. Royal Melbourne Hospital, Building 21, Royal Park Campus, 34-54 Poplar Road, Parkville, Victoria 3052, Australia.
E-mail address: Bhasker.Amatya@mh.org.au

2015, of the 5900 disasters worldwide, an estimated 3.2 billion people were affected and more than 1.2 million people lost their lives, with economic damage of around US$2 trillion.[3] In 2017 alone there were 318 natural disasters in 122 different countries, affecting 96 million people, with more than 9500 deaths and economic damage around US$ 314 billion.[4] Natural disasters occur disproportionately and regrettably, incapacitating impact is mostly shared by the low-resourced regions of the world,[5] accounting for more than 90% of deaths and 98% of people affected by natural disasters between 1991 and 2015.[6,7]

Current advancements in disaster response and management have improved survival rates of disaster victims, resulting in staggering number of people affected and/or injured, relative to fatalities (**Fig. 1**).[8–10] This includes a significant increase in the number of survivors with complex impairments and disability (temporary or permanent), from injuries, such as musculoskeletal (bone fractures, limb amputations, crush injuries), spinal cord injury (SCI), traumatic brain injury, soft tissue and peripheral nerve injury, and burns.[6,11–22] An increase in the number of people with exacerbation of chronic medical conditions (preexisting and/or new), psychological impairment, complications from initial injuries, and outbreaks of communicable diseases are frequently reported.[21–23] Further, people with preexisting disabilities are at higher risk of death and additional comorbidities/injuries. These signify integral role of comprehensive protracted rehabilitation not only to minimise trauma-related morbidity and mortality, but also to successfully reintegrate the survivors into community. The lack of such services leads to avoidable deaths, complications, long-term disability, and negative consequences to the individual, family and society at large.[14,21]

MEDICAL REHABILITATION DURING DISASTERS

The World Health Organization (WHO) defines rehabilitation as "a set of interventions designed to optimize function and reduce disability in individuals with health

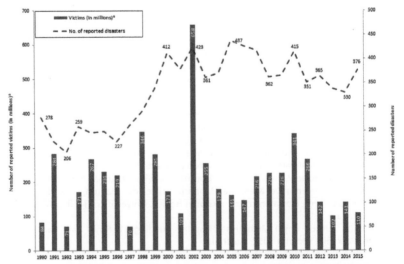

Fig. 1. Trends in occurrence and human impact of natural disaster (1990–2015). [a] Victims: sum of killed and total affected. (*From* Guha-Sapir D, Hoyois Ph, Below. R. Annual Disaster Statistical Review 2015: The Numbers and Trends. Brussels: CRED; 2016.)

conditions (disease, disorder, injury or trauma) in interaction with their environment."[24] The primary goals of medical rehabilitation are to address impairments and improve activity and participation within contextual factors (personal and environmental),[25] which align with the International Classification of Functioning, Disability and Health (ICF)[26] conceptual framework, whereby disability is understood as the result of the interaction of health condition and environmental factors.[27] Rehabilitation is a holistic approach to patient care delivered by an interdisciplinary team encompassing a range of professions, including (but not limited to) medical, physiotherapy, occupational therapy, orthotics and prosthetics, psychology, nutrition, and social work. The goals of rehabilitation in disaster settings are similar to any established rehabilitation setting, which include the management of injury and trauma, prevention and management of complications, enhancement and/or restoration of functional capabilities (including cognitive, neuropsychological function), prevention of permanent disability, and successful reintegration of survivors into the community.[21,25,27] However, in disaster settings, this process is more complex and challenging owing to different factors, such as a lack of skilled human resources (eg, rehabilitation physicians, allied health personnel), underdeveloped and/or limited access to local services, destruction and/or disruption of existing services, geophysical, communication, logistics, safety, sociocultural and other factors.[9,10,21,28,29]

In past disasters, despite a high prevalence of disaster-related disablement, most attention was on acute response plans/care protocols, which focus on saving lives and treating acute injuries, and rehabilitative needs were often neglected.[9,10,21,28] Often, there was insufficient rehabilitation capacity in the response planning, with negative consequences for affected individuals, families, and communities.[9,23,30] This was compounded by lack or inadequacy of rehabilitation services (still underdeveloped/not organized or absent) and a limited skilled clinical workforce in many low- and middle income countries, where most disasters occur, shifting the burden of rehabilitation to individuals (and their families).[9,20,28,31–33] According to the latest WHO data, in many of these low- and middle income countries the skilled rehabilitation practitioner density such as physiotherapists is less than 10 per 1 million population, and speech and occupational therapists, and rehabilitation physicians are very scarce or do not exist.[33] The situation is compounded in many large-scale disasters, when local health infrastructure (including rehabilitation resources) can be destroyed or disrupted, or be quickly overwhelmed by the influx of new victims.[20,21] A lack of access to timely comprehensive management, including rehabilitation, can further contribute to deteriorating preexisting inequality in health for these cohorts. On many occasions, many countries are reliant on international humanitarian assistance,[8] specifically on various types of emergency medical teams (EMTs).[23]

The global health authorities, including the WHO, emphasize that medical rehabilitation should be initiated acutely during the emergency disaster response and should be continued in the community over a longer-term.[10,21,34] The WHO World Report on Disability indicates that "rehabilitation services are essential services to be provided by foreign aid for humanitarian crises."[27(p108)] The Sphere Project, a voluntary initiative that sets common principles and universal minimum standards for the delivery of quality humanitarian response, in its handbook *Humanitarian Charter and Minimum Standards in Humanitarian Response*, further reinforces the importance of rehabilitation and states that surgery provided during a humanitarian crisis without any immediate rehabilitation can result in a failure in restoring functional capacity of the patient.[35]

726 Khan et al

Although need and demand of survivors can have different patterns in different emergencies, and may also differ over time,[23] rehabilitation is required at all phases of the disaster management continuum, which comprise the prevention, mitigation, preparation, response, and recovery phases.[10,20,21] Diagnostic, clinical management, educational, and advocacy capabilities of rehabilitation physicians are vital in disaster continuum phases. At times, rehabilitation physicians will be required to stretch beyond the roles they are trained for to meet the complex needs of the overwhelming number of disaster victims. Some of the potential roles of rehabilitation personnel in disaster management phases are presented in **Table 1**.

Table 1
Potential role of rehabilitation personnel in disaster continuum phases

Disaster Continuum Phases	Potential Role of Rehabilitation Personnel
Mitigation/ prevention	Raise public awareness Participation in disaster management planning and preparedness Participate/organize periodic evacuation and/or safety drills Training and education of health care professionals, community members and population at risk
Preparedness	All of above Participate in evacuation plans Coordination with the relevant stake-holders (both national and international) Establishment and development of survivors' management, triage, discharge, referral and tracking systems Development of guidelines, protocols, standards, etc.
Response	Participate in rescue activities Medical care and general health maintenance Postoperative care including prevention and management of complications Assessment of evolving and long-term injury patterns Rehabilitation needs and resource requirements (including provision of assistive devices) Patient education and self-care training (including carer and/or family) Referral to other services as required Establishment and planning of patient triage, discharge, referral, and tracking systems Collaboration with other rehabilitation and health care service providers, and coordination with emergency systems and local health system and government managers Education, training and capacity-building of local health care workforce
Recovery	Need assessment and long-term care and goal settings Evaluation of the level of disaster victims' social and occupational participation Assessment and modification of barriers to successful and efficient community reintegration Discharge planning and referral to other services as required Successful reintegration into the community Community rehabilitation, follow-up services and care continuum Vocational training and rehabilitation Participate in actions and activities to return the survivors to a safe environment Patient and carer education and training Seek financial assistance to the victims Data collection, management, and analysis

Fig. 2 indicates trends in the rehabilitation burden in sudden onset disasters (SODs) based on the time since the event and care needs of the affected population.[36] During acute disaster response, burden of rehabilitation in initial acute and evacuation stages are mainly due to influx of traumatic and nontraumatic emergencies; the burden increases in the postacute period as complications arise and survivors are prepared for triage to specialized facilities or discharge and in the longer term in the community for those with complex and permanent disabilities.[21,23,36] The demand for rehabilitation can increase over time, as triaging and discharging of patients (even those medically stable) can be problematic, owing to destruction or damage to their homes and livelihood. Further, demand for outpatient and community rehabilitation can increase after a disaster, creating additional resource and service needs.[23]

It is important to understand the nature of the disaster and its impact, ground situation, type of casualties, available resources, and potential burden of injuries/disease for the planning of any intervention. Further, the roles and responsibilities of the rehabilitation personnel can change as the disaster response progresses to reflect evolving clinical and rehabilitation needs.[21] The rehabilitation continuum model (**Fig. 3**) suggests a plan of rehabilitation intervention after a natural disaster, which includes a response phase based on individual clinical needs for acute and core rehabilitation stages (including community-based rehabilitation).[10,21] This model is based on assumptions of availability of rehabilitation services and workforce, and to our knowledge, is yet to be empirically tested.

CURRENT EVIDENCE OF REHABILITATION INTERVENTION IN DISASTER SETTINGS

Despite recognition of the critical importance of rehabilitation in natural disaster survivors, there is limited evidence owing to limited number of robust studies in

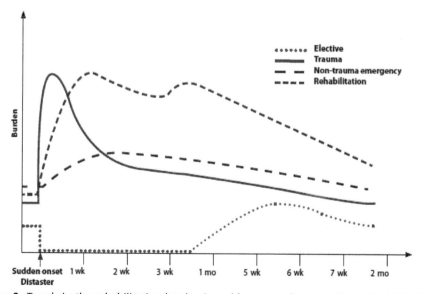

Fig. 2. Trends in the rehabilitation burden in sudden-onset disasters. (*From* World Health Organization. Emergency medical teams: minimum technical standards and recommendations for rehabilitation. Geneva: WHO; 2016; p. 13. Available at: https://extranet.who.int/emt/sites/default/files/MINIMUM%20TECHNICAL%20STANDARDS.pdf; with permission.)

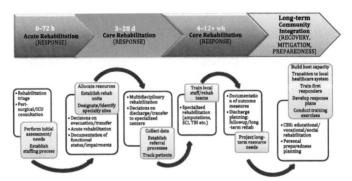

Fig. 3. Disaster continuum model. Unshaded = key clinical activities; shaded = nonclinical activities. (*Adapted from* Khan F, Amatya B, Gosney J, et al. Medical rehabilitation in natural disasters: a review. Arch Phys Med Rehabil 2015;96(9):1711; with permission.)

this area. This is reflected by various ethical, methodologic, and logistical challenges for researchers in disaster settings. The existing evidence highlights that early involvement of rehabilitation programs can reduce disability with better clinical outcomes, and improve participation and quality of life (QOL) of disaster survivors.[5,13,14] Published reports suggest that earthquake victims treated in centers with rehabilitation physician supervision have better clinical outcomes with fewer complications and a decreased length of hospital stay.[14,30] One comprehensive review evaluated the effectiveness of various medical rehabilitation interventions in natural disaster survivors.[10] The authors included 10 studies (2 randomized controlled trials and 8 observational studies) that investigated a variety of medical rehabilitation interventions for natural disaster survivors, ranging from comprehensive multidisciplinary rehabilitation to community educational programs. The interventions evaluated were heterogeneous and differed in many facets, including type, duration, intensity, and mode of delivery. However, the majority included physical activity and psychosocial intervention as rehabilitation components. The findings suggest evidence in favor of medical rehabilitation for survivors of natural disasters in producing short- and long-term gains for functional activities (activities of daily living, physical activity, etc), impairments (eg, psychological symptoms), and participation (QOL, social reintegration). The rehabilitation interventions were the strongest predictor of increased and sustained functional gains and improved health-related QOL. In China, a long-term structured and coordinated rehabilitation services NHV model (comprising nongovernmental organizations, local health departments, and volunteers) for earthquake survivors, significantly improved physical well-being. Further, psychological rehabilitation intervention (structured in-community psychological care) significantly improved psychosocial symptoms (post-traumatic stress disorder, depression, stress, etc) in post-tsunami victims. However, there was no evidence for the best type, mode, or intensity (frequency, duration) of these interventions or superiority of one intervention over another. **Table 2** provides summary of published studies evaluating various rehabilitation interventions in disaster settings.

THE WORLD HEALTH ORGANIZATION EMERGENCY MEDICAL TEAM INITIATIVE: A PARADIGM SHIFT

The international medical assistance effort (medical and surgical), collectively designated as an EMT (previously, Foreign Medical Team) have an integral role during

Table 2
Summary of rehabilitation interventions evaluated in disaster settings

References	Study Type	Interventions	Key Findings	Conclusion
Hospital-based rehabilitation program				
Hu et al,[37] 2012 China Disaster: 2008 Sichuan earthquake	Prospective cohort study N = 26 (SCI survivors)	Institution-based rehabilitation therapy (details not provided)	Significant improvement in functional status (ADLs, mobility, walking) Decrease in pain and depressive symptoms Significant improvement in QOL in the community ($P = .011$), self-ratings of QOL ($P<.001$), general health $P<.001$, and satisfaction with social relationships ($P = .017$) Improvement in physical health and psychological health improved (not statistically significant)	Significant improvements in: functional status, QOL, general health, satisfaction with social relationships and some areas of community integration (physical independence, mobility).
Li et al,[13] 2012 China Disaster: 2008 Sichuan earthquake	Prospective cohort study N = 51 (SCI survivors)	Individualized rehabilitation program provided by multidisciplinary rehabilitation team (rehabilitation physician, allied health therapists (PT, OT, traditional modalities), nurses, volunteers and other medical specialists)	35% patients achieved moderate ADLs independence and 90.2% regained self-care ability Rehabilitation program was the strongest predictor of significant increase in functional scores Earlier rescue and rehabilitation were significant positive predictors of rehabilitation effectiveness	Significantly improved functional rehabilitation outcomes with organized programs.

(continued on next page)

Table 2
(continued)

References	Study Type	Interventions	Key Findings	Conclusion
Li et al, 2015[38] China Disaster: 2008 Sichuan earthquake	Prospective cohort study N = 72 (amputees)	Institution-based rehabilitation to prevent joint contracture, desensitization, shaping of the residual limbs, joint mobilization, muscle strength training, PT, OT, and psychotherapy	Significant improvement in physical functioning ($P = .016$) and decrease in pain scores ($P<.001$) No significant changes in QOL or life satisfaction subscales Higher rates of literacy associated with better physical and mental health status Older age associated with decreased satisfaction with leisure activities and relationships	Significantly improved functioning and pain over time, however, no change in QOL and life satisfaction.
Ni et al,[39] 2013 China Disaster: 2008 Sichuan earthquake	Retrospective cohort study N = 450 survivors with fractures	Institution-based comprehensive rehabilitation program (therapeutic interventions, training/education, and vocational and social rehabilitation (details not provided)	Significant improvement in physical dysfunction ($P<.001$) Significant improvement in PTSD symptoms ($P<.05$) Female, average or above family income, having witnessed death and fearfulness were risk factors for PTSD symptoms, 50 mo after the earthquake	Physical dysfunction and PTSD were significantly decreased by rehabilitation intervention.

| Xiao et al,[16] 2011 China Disaster: 2008 Sichuan earthquake | Case series N = 174 survivors with tibial shaft fractures | Institution-based rehabilitation interventions delivered by physiotherapists | Functional recovery was positively associated with rehabilitation intervention (OR, 5.3; 95% CI, 2.38–11.67), but negatively correlated with the immobilization duration (OR, 0.87; 95% CI, 0.798–0.947), age (OR, [per 10-y increase] 0.54; 95% CI, 0.418–0.707), and depressive symptomatology (OR, 0.21; 95% CI, 0.063–0.716) | Functional recovery postrehabilitation of post-earthquake survivors with fractures. |
| Zhang et al,[17] 2012 China Disaster: 2008 Sichuan earthquake | Cross-sectional quasi-experimental study N = 390 survivors with fractures | Institutional-based rehabilitation (details not provided) | Significant improvement in ADLs and life satisfaction (P<.05) HRQOL improved more in early intervention subjects compared with controls (P = .008) Good performance of ADL (P<.001) and widowed marital status (P = .032) predicted high HRQOL, whereas pain was associated with worse outcomes (P<.001) Rehabilitation therapy, remunerative employment, and female gender were predictors of improved life satisfaction | Rehabilitation (early and late) significantly improved functional outcomes, HRQOL, and life satisfaction in earthquake fracture victims. |

(continued on next page)

Table 2
(continued)

Mixed (hospital- and community-based) rehabilitation model

References	Study Type	Interventions	Key Findings	Conclusion
Zhang et al,[40] 2013 China Disaster: 2008 Sichuan Earthquake	Longitudinal quasi-experimental study (3- arm) N = 510 Early intervention group (NHV-E): 298; late intervention group (NHV-L): 101 and control group: 111	NHV rehabilitation program comprised NGOs (N), local health departments (H), and professional rehabilitation volunteers (V): institutional-based rehabilitation followed by CBR	Significant improvement in physical functioning in the both early and late intervention groups Significant effects on spontaneous recovery	Significantly improved physical functioning of earthquake survivors

Psychological programs

References	Study Type	Interventions	Key Findings	Conclusion
Becker,[41] 2009 India Disaster: 2004 tsunami	Prospective cohort study N = 200	Community-based psychological program (group sessions)	Significant improvement in psychosocial symptoms IES scores: total ($P<.001$) and avoidance ($P<.001$), intrusion ($P<.001$), hypervigilance ($P<.001$)	Effective in reducing emotional distress for women tsunami survivors.
Berger and Gelkopf,[42] 2009 Sri Lanka Disaster: 2004 tsunami	Quasi-RCT with wait-list controls N = 166 elementary school students	School-based mental health program	Significant improvement in PTSD severity ($P<.001$), functional problems ($P<.001$), somatic complaints ($P<.001$), depression ($P<.001$), and hope ($P\leq.001$) scores	Helpful in mitigating post-disaster-related symptoms in children, and those with more severe symptoms benefited most.

Study	Study design	Intervention	Outcomes	Conclusions
Zhang et al,[43] 2013 China Disaster: 2008 Sichuan earthquake	RCT with wait-list controls N = 22	NET	Significant decreases in PTSD symptoms: avoidance, intrusion and hyperarousal subscales ($P<.001$ for all); anxiety and depression ($P<.001$), general mental stress ($P<.0001$) and increased post-traumatic growth ($P<.001$)	Significant positive effect on psychological symptoms and general mental health.
Social activity program				
Huang and Wong,[44] 2013 China Disaster: 2008 Wenchuan earthquake	Before and after qualitative study N = 24	Recreational activity groups	Participants' social networks broadened and strengthened Participant recognized the importance of mutual understanding and developed a sense of cooperation After participating in group activities, most women felt life was more meaningful or happy Participants' health improved	Effective in alleviating disaster survivors' feelings of distress and depression, improves their psychosocial well-being and recovery.

Abbreviations: ADLs, activities of daily living; CBR, community-based rehabilitation; CI, confidence interval; HRQOL, health-related quality of life; IES, impact of event scale; NET, narrative exposure therapy; NGOs, nongovernmental organizations; OR, odd ratio; OT, occupational therapist; PT, physiotherapist; PTSD, post-traumatic stress disorder; RCT, randomized, controlled trial.

Data from Khan F, Amatya B, Gosney J, et al. Medical rehabilitation in natural disasters: a review. Arch Phys Med Rehabil 2015;96(9):1709-27.

disasters and humanitarian crises. In many past disasters, international disaster relief was decided by the individual countries/or organizations, and teams often worked in silos, and on many occasions deployment was not always based on the needs of the situation.[45,46] There was lack of proper accreditation and/or coordination mechanism, and internal quality performance, and significant variation in capacities, competencies, and professional ethics.[46] In many disasters, there was huge influx of EMTs, which presented challenges to host country or disaster management authorities regarding coordination, management, and evaluation, resulting in inadequate care delivery, with often devastating consequences for the affected individuals, families, and communities.[9,21,23] For example, international humanitarian response to 2010 earthquake in Haiti (one of most deadliest earthquakes with over 316,000 people killed, 300,000 injured, and 1.3 million displaced) was catastrophic. There was influx of a large number of EMTs, with 44 deployed in the first month alone,[47] many were unregistered, and without standardized protocol, or coordination mechanisms in place.[46,48,49] Of those deployed, only 25% of EMTs adhered to essential deployment requirements and none followed the full requirements of the WHO and/or Pan American Health Organization.[50,51] There was poor coordination and communication, particularly between service providers (including EMTs), resulting in unsatisfactory outcomes and ineffective care delivery.[47,48,50,52] Reports suggest that a significant proportion of deaths that occurred in the days or weeks after the Haiti earthquake could have been prevented by improved patient care. Similarly, the number of EMTs deployed during the 2004 Indian Ocean tsunami exceeded demand.[46] EMTs specifically worked in silos, without coordination or standard frameworks.[51,53] These examples cautioned the international medical community to address these shortcomings and requirements for a stringent approach to emergency response in future disasters.[51,54] There is also increased scrutiny of the humanitarian sector and a drive toward professionalism and accountability.[55] The WHO's EMT initiative, one of the crucial developments in disaster management, follows a more systematic approach to medical team registration, deployment, and response coordination to natural disasters. For example, leadership of EMT initiative demonstrated efficacious coordination and management in typhoon Haiyan in the Philippines in 2013, tropical cyclone Pam in the Pacific region in 2015, the Nepal earthquakes in 2015, and others.[48] Various reports and guidelines are now published, one of the key being *Classification and Minimum Standards for Foreign Medical Teams in SODs*, published in September 2013.[52] This document set out benchmark requirements and standard for all EMTs seeking to respond to disasters and classifies all medical teams according to their capability into 3 main types (**Table 3**).[52]

The WHO EMT registration system, initiated in July 2015, enables the establishment of a global registry of EMTs for deployment in emergencies.[48] This EMT register will assist organizations in identifying suitable teams (country specific) when planning their responses in future disasters. To date, 22 acute medical teams (type 1 = 7, type 2 = 12, type 3 = 2 and 1 specialized cells) from different parts of the world have progressed to full verification and more than 75 teams have commenced the mentorship and quality assurance process.[48] However, currently no rehabilitation specialized cells are included in this list.

The EMT initiative currently comprises 11 working groups, including a rehabilitation group. The WHO-EMT initiative acknowledges rehabilitation as an integral aspect of medical response and patient-centered care in disaster settings,[52] and highlights that "rehabilitation is one of the core component of regular health care and, as such, all EMTs (both national and international) should have specific

Table 3
The WHO classification of EMTs

Type	Description	Capacity (per day)	Minimum Length of Stay (wk)
1 (Mobile)	Mobile outpatient teams: teams to access the smallest communities in remote areas	Over 50 outpatients	2
1 (Fixed)	Outpatient facilities with or without tented structure	Over 100 outpatients	2
2	Inpatient facilities with surgery	Over 100 outpatients and 20 inpatients; 7 major or 15 minor operations	3
3	Referral leave care, inpatient facilities, surgery and high dependency	Over 100 outpatients and 40 inpatients, including 4–6 intensive care beds; 15 major and 30 minor operations	4–6
Specialized care team[a]	Teams that can join local facilities or EMTs to provide supplementary specialist care for example, rehabilitation	Variable	Variable

[a] Specialize in a specific medical area, such as rehabilitation. May be as small 2 to 3 senior specialists, or a specialist facility.
From World Health Organization. Emergency medical teams: minimum technical standards and recommendations for rehabilitation. Geneva: WHO; 2016; p. 7. Available at: https://extranet.who.int/emt/sites/default/files/MINIMUM%20TECHNICAL%20STANDARDS.pdf; with permission.

and coordinated medical response plans for the provision of rehabilitation services to their patients for positive functional outcomes."[23,52] At the 2016 EMT Global Meeting in Hong Kong, first guideline for rehabilitation teams in SODs: the *Emergency medical teams: minimum technical standards and recommendations for rehabilitation* was launched.[23] This guideline is a collaborative product of the WHO, the International Society of Physical and Rehabilitation Medicine (ISPRM), and global rehabilitation experts,[23] and clearly sets out the core standards for rehabilitation services in SODs, regarding workforce, working areas, equipment/consumables, information management, and so on. It emphasizes building or strengthening the capacity of EMTs for rehabilitation for improved patient care and continuum of care beyond their departure from the affected area. The key minimum standards for EMTs include[23]:

- One or more rehabilitation professional per 20 beds at time of initial deployment, with further recruitment depending on case-load and local rehabilitation capacity.
- Allocation of specific rehabilitation space of at least 12 m^2 for all type 3 EMTs.
- Provision of essential rehabilitation equipment and consumables.

It is a requirement that all EMTs comply and adhere to these minimum technical standards.[23] The rehabilitation professionals as specialized care teams can either be integrated with other EMTs or into a local facility to augment their rehabilitation capacity.[23] The specialized teams are deployed at the request of ministry of health or coordinating cell of the host country and should comply with the same guiding principles and minimum core standards as EMTs (**Table 4**).

The guidelines also provide an overview of rehabilitation input and specific discharge considerations for common disaster-related injuries and to those with preexisting disability (**Table 5**). It emphasizes the importance of strengthening the local rehabilitation capacity to sustain care after the departure of the EMTs.[23] The rehabilitation professional should consider the appropriate referral pathway in accordance with the practices of the host country for all victims, specifically those requiring longer term care or with special needs, as early as possible (**Fig. 4**).

Table 4
Summary of technical standards for rehabilitation specialized team

	Minimum Technical Standards	Requirements for Verification
Team configuration	Team should be composed of ≥3 rehabilitation professionals, should be multidisciplinary and include at least 1 PT and other rehabilitation discipline(s): OT, rehabilitation physician, nurse, others.	Team can provide a list >3 professionals representing at least 2 rehabilitation disciplines (one of which is PT), who are available for rapid deployment.
Qualification and experience	Rehabilitation professionals should have at least a bachelor's degree or equivalent in their respective discipline and ≥3 y experience in trauma injury rehabilitation; ≥1 team member (preferably the team leader) should have experience in emergency response and all team members should have undergone training in working in austere environments.	Team can provide copies of professional qualifications and declarations of ≥3 y clinical experience in trauma injury rehabilitation.
Rehabilitation equipment[a]	Team should have capability to rapidly provide necessary equipment for deployment.	Team can present either a stockpile of the rehabilitation equipment, or documentation of an arrangement to have the equipment rapidly provided (including financial and logistical capability) in the event of the team's deployment.
Length of stay	Team that embeds into an EMT should stay for the minimum length of stay of that EMT (3 wk for a type II; 4–6 wk for a type III). A team that embeds into a local facility should plan to stay for ≥1 mo.	Team should declare its intended length of stay (not <3 wk), to facilitate appropriate placement with an EMT or local facility if deployed.

Abbreviations: OT, occupational therapists; PT, physiotherapists.
  [a] List of rehabilitation equipment is detailed in the guidelines (source: https://extranet.who.int/emt/guidelines-and-publications).
  Data from World Health Organization. Emergency medical teams: minimum technical standards and recommendations for rehabilitation. Geneva: WHO; 2016. Available at: https://extranet.who.int/emt/sites/default/files/MINIMUM%20TECHNICAL%20STANDARDS.pdf.

Table 5
Overview of rehabilitation input for common disaster-related injuries

Injury Type	Management Plan	Referral and Discharge Consideration
Basic fracture (conservative management)	Provide clear guidance on weight-bearing status Provide assistive devices Advise on ROM and functional use	Rehabilitation follow-up
Complex fracture	Provide assistive devices Advise on ROM and precautions Functional retraining External-fixator care Pain management Patient and care provider education Stabilize and refer according to national protocol or specialized care team/facility (if indicated)	Clarify time for removal of external fixator Progression of weight-bearing status Education about possible complications Rehabilitation follow-up
SCI	Neurologic assessment Pain management Functional retraining Provide temporary wheelchair Patient and care provider education and advice regarding pressure area prevention and care Refer according to national protocol or specialized care team/facility	Provide temporary assistive devices, including pressure-relieving equipment Educated on self-care, including bladder/bowel management and precautions Referral to local provider for long-term assistive devices Rehabilitation follow-up
Burns	Advise on appropriate dressing Positioning, including splinting if indicated ROM, strength, and functional retraining Patient and care provider education Refer to burns/plastics specialized care team/facility if indicated	Identify step-down facility if required Identify providers of local burns/plastics care and/or specialized burns care team for scar management, including compression garments Long-term rehabilitation follow-up required for scar maturation and risk for contracture

(continued on next page)

Table 5
(continued)

Injury Type	Management Plan	Referral and Discharge Consideration
Peripheral nerve injury	Positioning, including splinting if indicated Patient and care provider education ROM, strength, and functional retraining Pain management Refer to microsurgery specialized care team/facility if indicated	Identify microsurgery specialist care early if surgical intervention anticipated Referral to local provider for long-term assistive devices (such as orthotics) Education about possible complications, such as contracture Rehabilitation follow-up
Traumatic brain injury	Neurologic and cognitive assessments Positioning, including splinting if indicated ROM, strength, and functional retraining Patient and care provider education Refer to neurologic specialized care team/facility if indicated	Identify step-down facility if required Identify local providers of neurologic rehabilitation Provide long-term follow-up throughout neurologic recovery Referral to local provider for long-term assistive devices if indicated
Wounds	Advise on appropriate dressing Provide assistive devices ROM, strength, and functional retraining Patient and care provider education Refer to plastics specialized care team/facility if indicated	Identify plastics specialized care team early Progression of weight-bearing status Education about possible complications, such as infection Rehabilitation follow-up if indicated
Amputation	Preoperative advice according to prosthetic availability and functional outcomes Stump management Basic wound management Provide temporary assistive devices Pain management ROM, strength and functional retraining Patient and care provider education Refer according to national protocol or orthopedic specialized care team/facility	Referral to local provider for long-term assistive devices, such as prosthetic and/or wheelchair if indicated Rehabilitation follow-up

Abbreviation: ROM, range of motion.

From World Health Organization. Emergency medical teams: minimum technical standards and recommendations for rehabilitation. Geneva: WHO; 2016; p. 40-1. Available at: https://extranet.who.int/emt/sites/default/files/MINIMUM%20TECHNICAL%20STANDARDS.pdf; with permission.

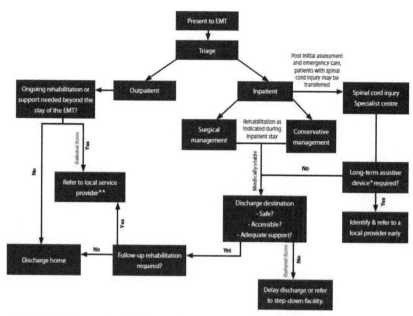

Fig. 4. Rehabilitation referral pathway for EMTs. * Such as prosthesis and orthosis or wheelchair; ** National facility, International Organization or Non-Governmental Organization. (*From* World Health Organization. Emergency medical teams: minimum technical standards and recommendations for rehabilitation. Geneva: WHO; 2016; p. 27. Available at: https://extranet.who.int/emt/sites/default/files/MINIMUM%20TECHNICAL%20STANDARDS.pdf; with permission.)

DISCUSSION

The WHO World Report on Disability strongly advocates that all Member States "develop, implement, and monitor polices, regulatory mechanisms, and standards for rehabilitation services, as well as promoting access to those services."[27(p122)] Further, the WHO Global Disability Action Plan 2014 to 2021 (Objective 2) emphasizes: "to strengthen and extend rehabilitation, rehabilitation, assistive technology, assistance and support services, and community-based rehabilitation."[56(p3)] There is evidence and consensus among international disaster management authorities that medical rehabilitation is an integral part of disaster management and improves survival, minimizes morbidity/complications and accelerates recovery, and also can maximize survivors' function, societal participation, and QOL.[5,9,10,20,21,23] However, in past disasters, the disaster response system largely focused on saving lives and management of acute injuries, with little regard for rehabilitative needs. There remain immense challenges, specifically for rehabilitation professionals, to respond promptly to the needs of people affected in disaster settings, because rehabilitation has been a low priority for many governments in majority of disaster-prone countries.[21,57] Many do not have an adequate rehabilitation-inclusive disaster management plan and/or much needed infrastructure and/or human resources, resulting in a shift of the burden of rehabilitation to survivors (families) and society. The WHO advocates all member states to develop partnerships to strengthen and extend high-quality, affordable rehabilitation services so that they can better respond to the needs of populations in its "Rehabilitation 2030: A Call for Action."[58] This call is further reaffirmed in the recent guideline, "Rehabilitation in Health Systems," which strongly recommends that rehabilitation services should be integrated into and between primary, secondary, and tertiary levels of health system of every country.[24]

The role of a rehabilitation professional is challenging, multidimensional, and reflects evolving clinical requirements, transitioning from emergency surgical support in established facilities to less acute rehabilitative input for injuries and complications in the community.[6,23] Rehabilitation professionals are experts in the diagnosis and treatment of general health conditions, and also in determining the prognosis of disability and functioning.[6] In any disaster setting, rehabilitation professional needs to be able to manage a wide spectrum of injuries (such as complex trauma, crushed injuries, fractures, burns, SCI, traumatic brain injury) and chronic conditions, and also work with (and train and educate) local health care providers to support community-based rehabilitation efforts for a continuum of care (such as prescription and use of assistive devices, mobility aids, and adaptive technologies).[9,20] Further, rehabilitation has a pivotal role in the education of survivors (and families) to cope with and adapt to acquired injury and disablement for reintegration into community. The absence and/or inadequacy of such services may lead to prolonged institutionalization and burden to society and health care system.

Effective delivery of rehabilitation care in disasters is challenging. The WHO's EMT guidelines mandate core standards for service delivery (including rehabilitation), for all disaster responders to ensure quick, and efficient care of survivors.[23,52] The key aims of the EMTs are to support and enhance local health care efforts and services and build the local capacity by educating/training local workforce. However, the WHO rehabilitation guidelines are yet to be implemented and EMT verification and registration process is complex, requiring substantial time and resources.[45] There is still uncertainty regarding the process of verifying specialized rehabilitation teams or embedding teams with larger verified EMTs, resulting in no verification of any rehabilitation team as an EMT or specialized team to date. Further, an exploration of previously identified needs, such as safety, security, logistical and operational issues during deployment, standardized education and training programs, standardized core competencies of EMTs, development of standardized tools (assessment, goal setting, evaluation, discharge/referral, etc), and resources for data collection, management, and dissemination are needed.[59,60]

Although local country capacity building of rehabilitation continues, as natural disasters escalate, there is likely need for international medical assistance (and humanitarian aid). Depending on the disaster type, magnitude, and setting, the need for EMTs (including rehabilitation professionals) will vary, as will the length of deployment. Therefore, response priorities and resource allocation should be aligned with local needs and disaster type. Knowledge and understanding of the crucial role of rehabilitation professionals among the policymakers and other health care professionals is essential.

THE WAY FORWARD

The WHO-EMT initiative is a paradigm shift in development of rehabilitation-inclusive disaster management.[52] The rehabilitation community needs to be resilient with leadership role of the WHO and ISPRM, and involvement of multi-stakeholder partnerships.[61] The ISPRM Disaster Rehabilitation Committee (DRC; formed in accordance with WHO-ISPRM Liaison initiative), advocates for the role of rehabilitation medicine in minimizing disability and optimizing functioning and health-related QOL in disasters.[21,62] The ISPRM DRC actively supports the WHO-EMT initiative, has contributed to developing the rehabilitation minimum standard guidelines, and in a process of creation of a central register/database of rehabilitation physicians from its more than 4000 members from

75 National Societies of Rehabilitation Medicine. These may in the future serve as a repository to facilitate the deployment of rehabilitation professionals in future disasters.[62] The DRC focuses on strengthening and capacity building of local rehabilitation service providers, including the development of rehabilitation infrastructure; training, education, or upskilling of local health personnel; and the strengthening of sustainable rehabilitation programs (community based, vocational) for long-term care. It has set up Specific Working Groups to oversee the DRC Action Plan, in particular an ISPRM response to deployment of rehabilitation physicians, to future disaster, if requested by the WHO and/or host disaster country (currently under review). Other activities include development of evidence-based guidelines and protocols for common disaster-related injuries, an on-line educational/training module, conducting a disaster-preparedness survey of rehabilitation physicians, and the development of standardized assessment tool for disaster settings. The ISPRM is involved in the mapping and evaluation of current rehabilitation facilities and personnel as well as emergency preparedness by the local authorities (particularly in disaster-prone regions) and upgrading the potential of these services for future disasters, if required.

Lessons learned from previous disasters and the incorporation of this information into long-term planning may serve to preclude repetition of mistakes made in past and decrease future vulnerability. Successful strategic implementation requires exhaustive context and situation analysis, because resource requirements may vary for each disaster. There is a need for investment in disaster risk reduction, planning and management with strong governance from relevant international and national bodies. Underlying factors of disaster risk such as poverty, climate change, rapid urbanization, environmental degradation, population growth, and others need to be considered.

Standard operating procedures on most common injuries or conditions based on clinical evidence-based standards in disaster settings are still lacking and the development of such standard operating procedures will facilitate and progress uniformity of quality of care. Standardized assessment and monitoring tools are yet to be developed, which can be challenging in terms of patient assessment and/or program monitoring and evaluation. There is lack of or insufficient population data in many disasters, which hinders identification of target population and/or deliver targeted interventions. Further, the absence of a platform for sharing and collection of data and/or research findings impedes planning and outcomes of care delivered, the provision and access to rehabilitation (and assistive technology), sustainable infrastructure, support services and education/research.[56]

In the future, the use of innovative models of rehabilitation (eg, mobile apps, telerehabilitation, mobile clinics, etc) can be a complementary approach to delivering timely, cost-efficient and patient-centered services, specifically in more remote areas. There is a need to increase public awareness and education about disability and rehabilitation.

IMPLICATIONS FOR CLINICAL PRACTICE

Rehabilitation clinicians play a significant role in disaster settings and can be key experts in the transition of patient care from the acute setting to the community. Depending on the scale and nature of disasters, the needs and challenges for rehabilitation might vary considerably. The recommendation for rehabilitation personnel (working independently in a specialized rehabilitation cell or embedded within other EMTs) include a proactive assessment and screening of disaster victims for common disaster-related problems and/or preexisting disability and medical conditions, regular specialist evaluation, and follow-up to assess need for appropriate intervention. The aim is to provide appropriate and adequate care to the disaster survivors, to achieve and maintain optimal functioning and independence, and successful reintegration into the community.

In any disaster, rehabilitation physicians need to act promptly and effectively with limited resources. Owing to the complexity and nature of injuries, rehabilitation programs should be individualized to meet the needs of patients. Further, the needs of disaster victims can be complex and cross physical, psychosocial, vocational, and other domains, requiring diverse modalities and interdisciplinary input with active patient and/or family participation. Specialized rehabilitation skills become increasingly necessary at times owing to the broad range of injuries and conditions of the victims. Their roles are indisputably multifaceted (from clinicians to the administrators) and are well-placed to address various challenges that arise during the complex disaster situations. There is growing evidence that chronic disease and long-term disability create great burden during and aftermath of disaster. However, current reporting of these issues is mostly anecdotal, with limited information and knowledge. All health professionals (including rehabilitation clinicians) should be aware of the potential difficulties and clinical needs of older adults, persons with preexisting disabilities and medical conditions, pregnant women, and children in a natural disaster, especially when evacuations and relocations occur.

IMPLICATIONS FOR RESEARCH

Disaster health research encompasses the traditional disaster cycle comprising the preparedness, response, recovery, and mitigation phases.[11] Health-related research must form an integral part of disaster response, to identify effective ways of mitigating the health impact of disasters and strengthen evidence base for interventions.[63] Conducting research in an emergency response situation is complex and challenging, because it poses ethical, methodologic, and logistical challenges for researchers.[64] It is further compounded by the limited importance of research process and lack of systems on acquiring data or integrating data into health information systems. Time for planning, ethical review processes, and resources may be in short supply in disaster settings.[64,65] Further distinctive features of ethical challenges of disaster research might include the following: populations affected by disaster may be traumatized and highly vulnerable to participate, research activities may hinder relief efforts, risks associated with research participation may shift rapidly as postdisaster situations evolve, and research protocols may be time-sensitive and need to be implemented quickly after a disaster event.[64] Participants may confuse research activities with relief operations; the potential population may not be able to provide consent or participate owing to language barrier or lack of education, or lack of family members and carers.[64] Ideally, research needs to be planned ahead and research ethics committees must develop procedures to ensure appropriate, timely, and flexible mechanisms and procedures (such as the prescreening of study protocols, advance and/or accelerated review) for ethical review and oversight.[63,64]

Research in disaster settings, particularly from the rehabilitation perspective, is scarce and specific evidence gaps exist for many rehabilitation interventions. There is need for robust research on the effectiveness and/or feasibility of specific rehabilitation interventions and to determine appropriate settings, target population, cultural and contextual considerations, and cost and safety. Further, there is a need for system-level research, including the types and impact of different service delivery models, governance structures, financial allocation, and distribution.[24] Mental health problems including posttraumatic stress disorder, depression, and anxiety are prevalent in all types of disasters and not well-studied. Research using reliable, valid, and user-friendly standardized tools (which reflects domains of the ICF framework) is needed. Further, development of specific indicators to measure the impact of implementation of the WHO guidelines is a priority. Overall, an iterative research process with multiple stakeholder partnership (embedded within new and existing systems) for monitoring and evaluation needs to be developed in future humanitarian endeavors.[55]

More rigorous research will improve the quality of evidence for different rehabilitation interventions in various disaster contexts.

SUMMARY

Recent advances in disaster response and rescue and field management have improved the survival rates of disaster victims significantly, resulting in an upsurge in survivors with complex and long-term disabling injuries. Many require comprehensive long-term interdisciplinary management, including rehabilitation, to restore their function and independence and maximize QOL. The critical importance and efficacy of rehabilitation services for survivors during and after a natural disaster is well-documented. Medical rehabilitation should be initiated in the immediate emergency response phase and should be included in the continuum of care over the longer term until treatment goals are achieved and survivors are successfully reintegrated into the society. The WHO rehabilitation guidelines recommend the implementation of and access to rehabilitation during all phases of disaster response and highlights rehabilitation as the longest and most costly phase of disaster management. Learning from past catastrophes, the WHO-EMT initiative and guidelines (including rehabilitation) are significant development in this area, which now provide structure and standardization aligned with principles to prepare for, plan, and provide comprehensive care during disasters. These developments are the much-needed steps in the right direction; however, there remain many challenges to implementing these standards. The key challenge ahead is to develop an integrated rehabilitation-inclusive approach to disaster planning and management, adapted to local needs. The delivery of timely, effective, patient-centered, coordinated, cost-efficient, and transparent services in future disasters is needed. The inclusion of rehabilitation physicians into either existing EMTs or as specialized cells is a priority. Future successful and effective disaster management will depend on the proficient leadership of the governing bodies, and the willingness and commitment of countries to build a systematic advance planning and preparedness to ensure that effective services, including rehabilitation are available in future disasters.

REFERENCES

1. Vos F, Rodriguez J, Below R, et al. Annual disaster statistical review 2009: the numbers and trends. Brussels (Belgium): Centre for Research on the Epidemiology of Disasters (CRED); 2010.
2. MICRODIS Health Working Group. PART I: literature review: health impact of natural disasters (earthquakes, windstorms and floods). Brussels (Belgium): MICRODIS; 2008.
3. Guha-Sapir D, Vanderveken A. CRED CRUNCH: the EM-DAT higher resolution disaster data (Issue No. 43). Brussels (Belgium): Centre for Research on the Epidemiology of Disasters (CRED); 2016.
4. Wallemacq P. CRED CRUNCH: natural disasters in 2017: lower mortality, higher cost (Issue No. 50). Brussels (Belgium): Centre for Research on the Epidemiology of Disasters (CRED); 2018.

5. Khan F, Amatya B, Rathore FA, et al. Medical rehabilitation in natural disasters in the Asia-Pacific region: the way forward. Int J Natural Disaster Health Secur 2015; 2(2):6–12.

6. Gosney J, Reinhardt JD, Haig AJ, et al. Developing post-disaster physical rehabilitation: role of the World Health Organization Liaison Sub-Committee on Rehabilitation Disaster Relief of the International Society of Physical and Rehabilitation Medicine. J Rehabil Med 2011;43(11):965–8.

7. United Nations International Strategy for Disaster Reduction. Natural Disasters and Sustainable Development: understanding the links between development, environment and natural disasters. Background Paper No. 5. Geneva (Switzerland): United Nations Department of Economic and Social Affairs; 2001.

8. Centre for Research on the Epidemiology of Disasters (CRED). The human cost of natural disasters: a global perspective. Brussels (Belgium): CRED; 2015.

9. Reinhardt JD, Li J, Gosney J, et al. Disability and health-related rehabilitation in international disaster relief. Glob Health Action 2011;4:7191.

10. Khan F, Amatya B, Gosney J, et al. Medical rehabilitation in natural disasters: a review. Arch Phys Med Rehabil 2015;96(9):1709–27.

11. Burns AS, O'Connell C, Rathore F. Meeting the challenges of spinal cord injury care following sudden onset disaster: lessons learned. J Rehabil Med 2012; 44(5):414–20.

12. Khan F, Amatya B, Dhakal R, et al. Rehabilitation needs assessment in persons following spinal cord injury in disaster settings: lessons learnt in 2015 Nepal earthquakes. Int J Phys Med Rehabil 2015;3:316.

13. Li Y, Reinhardt JD, Gosney JE, et al. Evaluation of functional outcomes of physical rehabilitation and medical complications in spinal cord injury victims of the Sichuan earthquake. J Rehabil Med 2012;44(7):534–40.

14. Rathore FA, Farooq F, Muzammil S, et al. Spinal cord injury management and rehabilitation: highlights and shortcomings from the 2005 earthquake in Pakistan. Arch Phys Med Rehabil 2008;89(3):579–85.

15. Rathore FA, Gosney J. Rehabilitation lessons from the 2005 Pakistan earthquake and others since - looking back and ahead? J Pak Med Assoc 2015;65(10): 1036–8.

16. Xiao M, Li J, Zhang X, et al. Factors affecting functional outcome of Sichuan-earthquake survivors with tibial shaft fractures: a follow-up study. J Rehabil Med 2011;43(6):515–20.

17. Zhang X, Hu XR, Reinhardt JD, et al. Functional outcomes and health-related quality of life in fracture victims 27 months after the Sichuan earthquake. J Rehabil Med 2012;44(3):206–9.

18. Landry MD, Singh CS, Carnie L, et al. Spinal cord injury rehabilitation in post-earthquake Haiti: the critical role for non-governmental organisations. Physiotherapy 2010;96(4):267–8.

19. Rathore MFA, Rashid P, Butt AW, et al. Epidemiology of spinal cord injuries in the 2005 Pakistan earthquake. Spinal Cord 2007;45(10):658–63.

20. Gosney JE Jr. Physical medicine and rehabilitation: critical role in disaster response. Disaster Med Public Health Prep 2010;4(2):110–2.

21. Rathore FA, Gosney JE, Reinhardt JD, et al. Medical rehabilitation after natural disasters: why, when, and how? Arch Phys Med Rehabil 2012;93(10):1875–81.

22. Handicap International and UK Emergency Medical Team. Rehabilitation in sudden onset disasters. London: Handicap International; 2015.

23. World Health Organization. Emergency medical teams: minimum technical standards and recommendations for rehabilitation. Geneva (Switzerland): WHO; 2016.
24. World Health Organization. Rehabilitation in health systems 2017. p. 2017. Geneva (Switzerland): WHO; 2017.
25. Khan F, Amatya B, Hoffman K. Systematic review of multidisciplinary rehabilitation in patients with multiple trauma. Br J Surg 2012;99(Suppl 1):88–96.
26. World Health Organization (WHO). International classification of functioning, disability and health (ICF). Geneva (Switzerland): WHO; 2001.
27. World Health Organization. World report on disability. Geneva (Switzerland): WHO; 2011.
28. Khan F, Amatya B, Mannan H, et al. Rehabilitation in Madagascar: challenges in implementing the World Health Organization disability action plan. J Rehabil Med 2015;47(8):688–96.
29. Smith E, Wasiak J, Sen A, et al. Three decades of disasters: a review of disaster-specific literature from 1977-2009. Prehosp Disaster Med 2009;24(4):306–11.
30. Mallick M, Aurakzai JK, Bile KM, et al. Large-scale physical disabilities and their management in the aftermath of the 2005 earthquake in Pakistan. East Mediterr Health J 2010;16(Suppl):S98–105.
31. Economic and Social Commission for Asia and the Pacific (ESCAP). Disasters in Asia Pacific: 2104 year in review. Bangkok (Thailand): United Nations; 2015.
32. Rathore FA, New PW, Iftikhar A. A report on disability and rehabilitation medicine in Pakistan: past, present, and future directions. Arch Phys Med Rehabil 2011; 92(1):161–6.
33. World Health Organization. The need to scale up rehabilitation: background paper (WHO/NMH/NVI/17.1). Geneva (Switzerland): WHO; 2017.
34. Landry MD, McGlynn M, Ng E, et al. Humanitarian response following the earthquake in Haiti: reflections on unprecedented need for rehabilitation. World Health Popul 2010;12(1):18–22.
35. The Sphere Project Team. In: Greaney P, Pfiffner S, Wilson D, editors. Humanitarian charter and minimum standards in humanitarian response. 3rd edition. Rugby (United Kingdom): Practical Action Publishing; 2011. p. 292–391.
36. von Schreeb J, Riddez L, Samnegard H, et al. Foreign field hospitals in the recent sudden-onset disasters in Iran, Haiti, Indonesia, and Pakistan. Prehosp Disaster Med 2008;23(2):144–51.
37. Hu X, Zhang X, Gosney JE, et al. Analysis of functional status, quality of life and community integration in earthquake survivors with spinal cord injury at hospital discharge and one-year follow-up in the community. J Rehabil Med 2012;44(3): 200–5.
38. Li L, Reinhardt JD, Zhang X, et al. Physical function, pain, quality of life and life satisfaction of amputees from the 2008 Sichuan earthquake: a prospective cohort study. J Rehabil Med 2015;47:466–71.
39. Ni J, Reinhardt JD, Zhang X, et al. Dysfunction and post-traumatic stress disorder in fracture victims 50 months after the Sichuan earthquake. PLoS One 2013;8(10): e77535.
40. Zhang X, Reinhardt JD, Gosney JE, et al. The NHV rehabilitation services program improves long-term physical functioning in survivors of the 2008 Sichuan earthquake: a longitudinal quasi experiment. PLoS One 2013;8(1):e53995.
41. Becker SM. Psychosocial care for women survivors of the tsunami disaster in India. Am J Public Health 2009;99(4):654–8.

42. Berger R, Gelkopf M. School-based intervention for the treatment of tsunami-related distress in children: a quasi-randomized controlled trial. Psychother Psychosom 2009;78(6):364–71.

43. Zang Y, Hunt N, Cox T. A randomised controlled pilot study: the effectiveness of narrative exposure therapy with adult survivors of the Sichuan earthquake. BMC Psychiatry 2013;13:41.

44. Huang Y, Wong H. Effects of social group work with survivors of the Wenchuan earthquake in a transitional community. Health Soc Care Community 2013; 21(3):327–37.

45. Amatya B, Galea M, Li J, et al. Medical rehabilitation in disaster relief: towards a new perspective. J Rehabil Med 2017;49(8):620–8.

46. Global Health Cluster - Foreign Medical Team Working Group. Registration and coordination of Foreign Medical Teams responding to sudden onset disasters: the way forward. Geneva (Switzerland): World Health Organization; 2013.

47. Tataryn M, Blanchet K. Evaluation of post-earthquake physical rehabilitation response in Haiti, 2010 – a systems analysis. London: International Centre for Evidence on Disability (ICED): London School of Hygiene & Tropical Medicine (LSHTM) (Funded by CBM); 2012.

48. World Health Organization. Emergency medical teams: World Health Organization EMT initiative. Geneva (Switzerland): WHO; 2016.

49. de Goyet CdV, Sarmiento J, Grünewald F. Health response to the earthquake in Haiti January 2010: lessons to be learned for the next massive sudden-onset disaster. Washington, DC: Pan American Health Organization (PAHO); 2011.

50. Gerdin M, Wladis A, von Schreeb J. Foreign field hospitals after the 2010 Haiti earthquake: how good were we? Emerg Med J 2013;30(1):e8.

51. Burkle FM Jr, Nickerson JW, von Schreeb J, et al. Emergency surgery data and documentation reporting forms for sudden-onset humanitarian crises, natural disasters and the existing burden of surgical disease. Prehosp Disaster Med 2012; 27(6):577–82.

52. Global Health Cluster - Foreign Medical Team Working Group. Classification and minimum standards for foreign medical teams in sudden onset disasters. Geneva (Switzerland): World Health Organization; 2013.

53. Lind K, Gerdin M, Wladis A, et al. Time for order in chaos! A health system framework for foreign medical teams in earthquakes. Prehosp Disaster Med 2012; 27(1):90–3.

54. Burkle FM Jr. The development of multidisciplinary core competencies: the first step in the professionalization of disaster medicine and public health preparedness on a global scale. Disaster Med Public Health Prep 2012;6(1):10–2.

55. Smith J, Roberts B, Knight A, et al. A systematic literature review of the quality of evidence for injury and rehabilitation interventions in humanitarian crises. Int J Public Health 2015;60(7):865–72.

56. World Health Organization. WHO global disability action plan 2014–2021: better health for all people with disability. Geneva (Switzerland): WHO; 2014.

57. Amatya B, Khan F. Overview of medical rehabilitation in natural disasters in the Pacific Island Countries. Phys Med Rehabil Int 2016;3(4):1090.

58. World Health Organization. Rehabilitation: key for health in the 21st century (WHO/NMH/NVI/17.3). Geneva (Switzerland): WHO; 2017.

59. Daily E, Padjen P, Birnbaum M. A review of competencies developed for disaster healthcare providers: limitations of current processes and applicability. Prehosp Disaster Med 2010;25(5):387–95.

60. Ripoll Gallardo A, Djalali A, Foletti M, et al. Core competencies in disaster management and humanitarian assistance: a systematic review. Disaster Med Public Health Prep 2015;9(4):430–9.
61. Stucki G, von Groote PM, DeLisa JA, et al. Chapter 6: the policy agenda of ISPRM. J Rehabil Med 2009;41(10):843–52.
62. International Society of Physical and Rehabilitation Medicine (ISPRM). Policy statement: response to a sudden-onset natural disaster. Geneva (Switzerland): ISPRM; 2016.
63. Council for International Organizations of Medical Sciences (CIOMS). Guideline 20: research in disaster situations. Geneva (Switzerland): CIOMS; 2013.
64. Hunt M, Tansey CM, Anderson J, et al. The challenge of timely, responsive and rigorous ethics review of disaster research: views of research ethics committee members. PLoS One 2016;11(6):e0157142.
65. Lee AC, Booth A, Challen K, et al. Disaster management in low- and middle-income countries: scoping review of the evidence base. Emerg Med J 2014; 31(e1):e78–83.

Physical Medicine and Rehabilitation in Latin America: Development and Current Status

Carolina Schiappacasse, MD[a], Juan Manuel Guzmán, MD[b],
Maria Herrera Dean, MD[c], Sandra Corletto, MD[d],
Linamara Rizzo Battistella, MD, PhD[e], Marta Imamura, MD[f],
Jorge Gutiérrez, MD[g], Graciela Borelli, MD[h], Diana Muzio, MD[i],
William Micheo, MD[j],*

KEYWORDS

- Physical medicine • Rehabilitation • Latin America • Education • Clinical activities

KEY POINTS

- Disability is a global health and human rights issue that leads to poor health outcomes, lower educational achievement, less economic participation, and has a higher incidence in low and middle income countries, which include many in Latin America.
- The specialty of Physical Medicine and Rehabilitation developed in the Latin American region as a medical field following the Second World War and the polio epidemic of the 1950s. Over the past 60 years it has increased its presence in the region, working to improve patient function and quality of life.

Continued

Disclosure: The authors have nothing to disclose.
[a] British Hospital, Clínica de Rehabilitación Las Araucarias, San Martin University, Buenos Aires, Argentina; [b] Physical Medicine and Rehabilitation, Electrodiagnostic and EMG, Mexican Academy of Surgery, Indiana # 260-808, Col. Napoles, Mexico City CP 03810, Mexico; [c] Gerente centro Especializado de Medicina Fisica y Rehabilitación, Instituto Hondureño de Seguridad Social, El Barrial. 7-8 ave. 3-4 Calle No. 7, San Pedro Sula, Honduras; [d] Centro de Rehabilitación y Electrodiagnostico CRE, Honduras; [e] University of Sao Paulo, School of Medicine, Clinical Hospital of USP, Sao Paulo, Brazil; [f] Departamento de Medicina Legal, Etica Medica e Medicina Social e do Trabalho, Faculdade de Medicina FMUSP, Universidade de Sao Paulo, Sao Paulo, Brazil; [g] Centro de Rehabilitación Potenciales, Calle 5 #38. 14 Suite 501, Cali Valle, Colombia; [h] Agregada de Rehabilitación y Medicina Física, Universidad de la República, Jose Enrique Rodo 1714 apto. 301, Montevideo, Uruguay; [i] Universidad de Medicina de Buenos Aires, Buenos Aires, Argentina; [j] Physical Medicine, Rehabilitation and Sports Medicine Department, University of Puerto Rico, School of Medicine, PO Box 365067, San Juan, PR 00936-5067, USA
* Corresponding author.
E-mail addresses: william.micheo@upr.edu; wmicheo@usa.net

Phys Med Rehabil Clin N Am 30 (2019) 749–755
https://doi.org/10.1016/j.pmr.2019.07.001
1047-9651/19/© 2019 Elsevier Inc. All rights reserved.

Continued

- There are many challenges and opportunities for the specialty of PM&R in the future, but with improved educational programs, evidence-based treatment strategies, higher research output, and better coverage of services, the specialty will continue to develop and expand to cover the needs of patients with disabling conditions in the Latin America.

INTRODUCTION

The world report on disability published by the World Health Organization (WHO) presented that 15% of the world population or 1 in 7 individuals suffers from disability and 2% to 4% have severe difficulties in functioning.[1] Disability disproportionally affects women, and older and poor people, in particular indigenous individuals and ethnic minorities. Disability is a global health and human rights issue that leads to poor health outcomes, lower educational achievement, and less economic participation and has a higher incidence in low and middle income countries, which include many in Latin America.[1,2] The WHO and the Pan-American Health Organization (PAHO) have established an action plan to address some of the causes of increasing disability, which include inadequate policies and funding, lack of provision of services, and difficulties with access to care.[3]

The PAHO defines rehabilitation as a set of interventions designed to optimize functioning and reduce disability in individuals with health conditions in interaction with their environment and recognizes rehabilitation as one of the essential services defined within universal health coverage.[4] The WHO recommends that rehabilitation should be integrated into health systems worldwide. Specific recommendations include that rehabilitation services should be integrated in primary, secondary, and tertiary levels of care, a multidisciplinary rehabilitation workforce should be available, community and hospital rehabilitation services should be offered, hospitals should include specialized rehabilitation units for inpatients with complex needs, financial resources should be allocated for rehabilitation, health insurance should cover rehabilitation services, and policies should ensure that assistive devices and training and their use are available to everyone who needs them.[5]

Physical Medicine and Rehabilitation (PM&R) and in some parts of the world Physical and Rehabilitation Medicine (PRM) is the medical specialty that manages disorders or disability of the muscles, bones, and the nervous system with goals of restoring function, reducing pain, and improving quality of life.[6] The specialty of PM&R developed in the Latin American region as a medical field following the Second World War and the polio epidemic of the 1950s. Over the past 60 years it has increased its presence in the region, working to improve patient function and quality of life. The development of graduate educational programs in the specialty, inpatient and outpatient rehabilitation services, and scientific progress in Rehabilitation Medicine have put the specialty in the forefront of addressing the needs of children and adults with disability or disabling illness.[7,8]

In this article, we present the history and current status of the specialty of PM&R in Latin America. We discuss issues related to education, clinical practice, future challenges, and opportunities that face the medical specialty of physiatry in the region. The authors represent different countries in Central and South America as well as the Caribbean, and the information presented is a combination of the limited number of articles published on the topic in the medical literature, information provided by the authors related to the practice of the specialty in their countries, and data gathered from a questionnaire sent to representatives of PM&R in different countries of the region.

HISTORY

Rehabilitation services have existed in Latin America since the beginning of the twentieth century. Countries such as Mexico had rehabilitation services that included hydrotherapy, mechanotherapy, and electrotherapy in the early 1900s.[9] Medical rehabilitation services originated in the 1940s, many under the leadership of orthopedic surgeons who identified a need to prevent and treat musculoskeletal problems following illness, injury, or surgical interventions. Argentina and Mexico developed physical medicine services in the 1940s, and in 1949 the Argentinian Society of Physical Medicine and Rehabilitation was established.[7] The specialty of PM&R originated in many countries in the 1950s, with hospitals and government institutions creating Physical Medicine and Rehabilitation departments.

Medical training programs in the specialty started as early as 1947 in Uruguay. Physicians from Colombia trained in the United States under Dr Howard Rusk and other specialists trained in Mexico and returned to their countries of origin to establish academic programs and clinical rehabilitation services. Formal graduate education programs in PM&R continued to develop in the decade of 1960 with residency training starting in Puerto Rico, Mexico, Colombia, and Argentina. In 1977, courses in Cardiac Rehabilitation and Electromyography were organized by Dr Juan Quintal Velasco in Mexico, and Dr Florencio Saez from Puerto Rico created the Puerto Rican Academy of Electrodiagnosis and Electromyography, providing training through clinical rotations and exchange programs to many specialists from different countries in Latin America.

Clinical practice expanded in the 1970s and included care of victims of polio, cerebral palsy, spinal cord injury, stroke, amputation, musculoskeletal conditions, and pain. In many countries, the initial rehabilitation efforts were toward children with disabling conditions; management of adults with disability developed at later stages, particularly following the Second World War.[7]

The Latin American Society of Physical Medicine and Rehabilitation (AMLAR) was founded in Mexico in 1961 with representatives of 13 countries in Central and South America and Puerto Rico; the first AMLAR congress took place in 1963. After the initial congress, the society has expanded to include 23 member countries and has organized 24 international scientific congresses in all regions of Latin America.

Rehabilitation services are covered through legislation in many countries of the region. Over the past 20 years, legislation has been passed for individuals with disability dealing with access to rehabilitation care, discrimination, and equal opportunity. Countries such as Argentina, Brazil, and Colombia have passed disability-related laws starting in the 1980s and have developed a national plan of rehabilitation including services in universal health care.[10]

EDUCATION

Training programs in PM&R have been developed in most countries in Central America, South America, and the Spanish-speaking islands of the Caribbean. There is a wide variety of training experiences and models of education in the region; however, over the past decade some standardization of training experiences has occurred. Most training is of 3 years' duration, with a growing number of institutions moving to 4 years of education. A small number of programs are of 5 years' duration.

Training experiences include inpatient and outpatient rehabilitation management, treatment of patients with complex rehabilitation issues, management of children, amputees, pain, and electrodiagnosis. Some countries such as Brazil, Mexico, and Puerto Rico offer subspecialty training in pain management, electro diagnostic medicine, sports medicine, pediatric rehabilitation, and neurologic rehabilitation.

Many programs offer training and protected time for research during residency. An increasing number require research projects, preparation of scientific manuscripts, or a research thesis before graduation. Residents are encouraged to present their research projects in local, regional, national, or international scientific meetings. The Mexican Society of PM&R established a national scientific program for rehabilitation residents in 2004, and awards the authors of the 3 best papers of the meeting the opportunity to publish the abstracts of their work in *PM&R*, the official journal of the American Academy of Physical Medicine and Rehabilitation.

Most funding for training is provided by government institutions, such as universities, social security services, and military hospitals, but some residency education is provided by private institutions. Most residents are trained in Mexico, Brazil, and Argentina (**Table 1**).

Some countries require an examination before becoming certified as a PM&R specialist. In others, specialists are recognized by a national board of specialists, national PM&R societies, or other government agencies. Argentina and Mexico have established maintenance of certification programs following graduation from residency.

Continued medical education for PM&R specialists in practice is provided by national, regional, and international PM&R professional societies. Many societies offer annual educational activities for its members and annual or biannual scientific congresses. AMLAR organizes an international congress every 2 years with invited speakers from many of the Latin American countries and experts from the United States and other regions of the world. The location and organization of this meeting is rotated throughout the Latin American region. The congress for 2018 took place in Guayaquil, Ecuador, and the next meeting will take place in La Paz, Bolivia, in 2020.

Cuba, Brazil, Mexico, Colombia, and Argentina, have peer-reviewed scientific journals in PM&R. Brazil's Journal Acta Fisiatrica is published in English, online with open

Table 1
List of physical medicine and rehabilitation residency training program and average number of residents per country

Country	Total Numbers of Residency Programs	Average Numbers of Residents in Training
Brazil	17	99
Argentina	19	104
Uruguay	1	24
Honduras	1	9–15
Peru	8	90
Colombia	6	95
Mexico	16	272
Cuba	1	179
Dominican Republic	2	17
Puerto Rico	2	24

access, and indexed LILACS and LATINDEX. Research activities and scientific publications have increased in the region, but this is an area that needs to be further developed.

CLINICAL PRACTICE

The number of PM&R specialists has grown significantly in Latin America over the past 2 decades, but this varies widely from country to country and the number of specialists is not sufficient to cover the needs of the region. The Mexican Institute for Social Security recommends a ratio of 1 PM&R specialist for every 100,000 inhabitants of a country, and most countries of the region do not reach this milestone (**Fig. 1**). The WHO, in its Rehabilitation 2030: a call to action meeting, recognized that although there has been an increase in rehabilitation professionals, which include PM&R physicians, there is still a big need for these services, particularly in poor countries, where the ratio of 10 rehabilitation professionals per 1,000,000 inhabitants is not achieved.[11] Another important issue is that PM&R services are concentrated around larger cities and metropolitan areas, with many rural, remote, and poor regions lacking services.

Many of the countries in the region have a national rehabilitation plan, and provide services through universal health coverage (**Table 2**). PM&R services are provided in primary, secondary, and tertiary levels of medical care. Mexico has developed a model of having rehabilitation services led by a PM&R specialist in family medicine centers, rehabilitation services at secondary government hospitals, and tertiary services at specialized rehabilitation centers.[8] Smaller countries like Honduras provide services in all 3 levels of medical attention, and many in the region are developing community-based rehabilitation to address needs of individuals with disabling conditions who live outside major metropolitan areas where access to more advanced rehabilitation and technology remains limited.

There has been a development in PM&R private services provided by institutions or individual practitioners. These vary from country to country and many rehabilitation services are not integrated. Areas of care that have expanded include pain medicine, sports medicine, neurologic rehabilitation including spasticity management, cardiac, vocational and geriatric rehabilitation and electrodiagnostic medicine. Over the past decade, there has been a significant interest in the use of newer diagnostic and

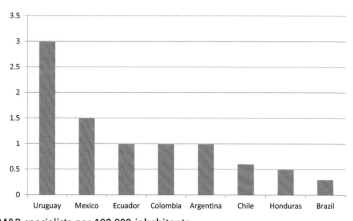

Fig. 1. PM&R specialists per 100,000 inhabitants.

| Table 2 |
| Countries with national rehabilitation plan and universal rehabilitation health coverage ||| |
Country	National Rehabilitation Plan	Universal Coverage
Brazil	Yes	Yes
Argentina	Yes	Yes
Honduras	No	No
Colombia	Yes	Yes
Mexico	Yes	Yes
Cuba	Yes	Yes
Puerto Rico	No	No

therapeutic approaches in the care of patients, which includes musculoskeletal ultrasound, regenerative techniques, and interventional pain management.

With an increased number of the older individuals with chronic diseases and disability, the need for rehabilitation services has increased. PM&R physicians are serving injured workers; motor vehicle accident and violence victims; neurologic patients with stroke, traumatic brain injury, and spinal cord injury; and patients with musculoskeletal problems and chronic pain.

CHALLENGES AND OPPORTUNITIES

The challenges to the specialty of PM&R are multiple, and include limited information on disability and disabling conditions in many countries of the region; difficulty in comparing models of provision of rehabilitation care across different countries; variation in official government policies regarding coverage of rehabilitation technology and treatments for different patient populations; lack of integration and fragmentation between public and private sectors in the provision of rehabilitation; poor coverage of services in rural areas; lack of continuum of treatments from primary and secondary to tertiary levels of care; and need for the development of better patterns of referral among the medical specialties involved in the care of patients with disabling conditions.

In terms of education, there is a need to improve postgraduate training, including the development of educational requirements and core competencies for the specialty, academic and clinical knowledge that needs to be achieved at the completion of training in order to enter independent medical practice, and an increase in scientific productivity of residents and faculty.

The opportunities for the specialty are many, including the development of a collaboration strategy between national rehabilitation societies and government organizations, AMLAR, the International Society of Physical and Rehabilitation Medicine Society, PAHO, and the WHO. This collaboration could result in unified standards in several areas, which include rehabilitation services for each level of clinical attention, clinical practice guidelines, clear parameters for accreditation of rehabilitation centers and medical services, development of rehabilitation information technology, postgraduate education across the countries in the region, and research development and infrastructure. Other areas of opportunity include improving access to care in rural areas by providing incentives to PM&R physicians and rehabilitation professionals to move to these regions, establishing stronger referral networks with other medical specialists, and increasing the number of PM&R specialists by developing additional training programs in countries in which these exist and creating new programs in Latin American countries without residency training.

SUMMARY

- There has been an increase in disability around the world, in particular affecting individuals in low to middle income countries, many which are located in Latin America.
- The medical specialty of PM&R is one of the latest specialties to develop in Latin America, exhibiting a significant growth over the past several decades.
- The development of training programs, expansion of clinical services, and increased scientific productivity have advanced the specialty in the region.
- Despite the growth of PM&R, there is a need to increase the number of specialists to manage disabling conditions, musculoskeletal injuries, and pain.
- There are many challenges and opportunities for the specialty of PM&R in the future, but with improved educational programs, evidence-based treatment strategies, higher research output, and better coverage of services, the specialty will continue to develop and expand to cover the needs of patients with disabling conditions in the Latin America.

REFERENCES

1. World Health Organization, The World Bank. World report on disability. Geneva (Switzerland): World Health organization; 2011.
2. Morgan Banks L, Kuper H, Polack S. Poverty and disability in low and middle-income countries: a systematic review. PLoS One 2017;12(20):e0189996.
3. WHO global disability action plan 2014-2021, "better health for all people with disability". Geneva (Switzerland): World Health Organization; 2015.
4. Available at: http://www.paho.org. Accessed November 1, 2018.
5. Rehabilitation in health systems. Geneva (Switzerland): World Health Organization; 2017.
6. Available at: http://www.abpmr.org. Accessed November 8, 2018.
7. Sotelano F. History of rehabilitation in Latin America. Am J Phys Med Rehabil 2011;91(4):368–73.
8. Available at: http://www.portalamlar.org. Accessed November 12, 2018.
9. Guzman-Gonzalez JM. Rehabilitation in Mexico: a dream come true. PM R 2012; 10:770–2.
10. Available at: http://cepal.org. Accessed November 12, 2018.
11. Rehabilitation 2030: a call to action. Geneva (Switzerland): World Health Organization; 2017.

Rehabilitation in Africa

Sisay Gizaw Geberemichael, MD[a],*,
Abena Yeboaa Tannor, BSc, MBChB, MSc (Rehab), MGCP[b],
Tesfaye Berhe Asegahegn, MD[a], Asare B. Christian, MD, MPH[c],
Gloria Vergara-Diaz, MD[d,1], Andrew J. Haig, MD[e,f,2]

KEYWORDS

- Rehabilitation • Rehabilitation services • Disability research • Africa
- Community-based rehabilitation

KEY POINTS

- Comprehensive rehabilitation services are inequitable or inaccessible in Africa.
- In Africa, the needs for multidisciplinary rehabilitation services are expected to continuously increase in the years to come.
- Along with working policies and delivery strategies, good governance practices help in addressing the increasing unmet needs for rehabilitation in Africa.
- Multisectoral and multistakeholder partnerships are required for efficient mobilization and utilization of rehabilitation resources in Africa.

INTRODUCTION

Despite the progress toward comprehensive multidisciplinary rehabilitation practices in Africa, a continent inhabited by 14% of the world population, shortages of resources and expertise for rehabilitation services and research continue.[1–5] These unmet needs for rehabilitation are likely to increase in the future with the recent trends of increasing prevalence of chronic illnesses and injuries and improving life expectancies in the continent.[1,5,6] Critical analysis of disability data, indigenous knowledge, and local contextual factors will undoubtedly lead to functional policy frameworks and delivery models for accessible and equitable rehabilitation services and assistive

Disclosure: The authors have nothing to disclose.
[a] Department of Neurology, St. Paul's Hospital Millennium Medical College, PO Box 1271, Addis Ababa, Ethiopia; [b] Disability and Rehabilitation Studies, Komfo Anokye Teaching Hospital, Kwame Nkrumah University of Science and Technology, PO Box: 1934, Kumasi, Ghana; [c] Good Shepherd Rehabilitation Hospital, PO Box: 850 South 5th Street, Allentown, PA 18103, USA; [d] Department of Physical Medicine and Rehabilitation, Harvard Medical School, Spaulding Rehabilitation Hospital, Boston, MA, USA; [e] The University of Michigan, Ann Arbor, MI, USA; [f] Haig Consulting PLC, MI, USA
[1] Present address: PO Box 300 First Avenue, Charlestown, MA 02129.
[2] Present address: PO Box: 524, Londonderry, VT 05148.
* Corresponding author. PO Box 12111, Addis Ababa, Ethiopia.
E-mail address: giz6sisay@live.com

Phys Med Rehabil Clin N Am 30 (2019) 757–768
https://doi.org/10.1016/j.pmr.2019.07.002
1047-9651/19/© 2019 Elsevier Inc. All rights reserved.

technologies.[1,7] Rehabilitation workforce training programs customized for local priorities and facilitation of interprofessional learning are relevant in building the capacities for locally inclusive disability and rehabilitation research, and good governance of high-quality comprehensive rehabilitation services in the continent.[1,7,8]

In this article, current status of rehabilitation services, multidisciplinary rehabilitation workforces, and availability and quality of rehabilitation and disability data in Africa are reviewed. The quest for adapted, locally sensitive and reflexive policies and service delivery models is discussed. Rehabilitation governance and leadership recommendations and strategies for human resource development also are explored. Moreover, guiding principles and potential dimensions for partnerships for local, regional, and international stakeholders in rehabilitation in Africa are highlighted.

DISABILITY AND REHABILITATION PRACTICES IN AFRICA

Africa, the second most populous continent with more than a billion largely rural (61%) dwellers, has recently seen economic growth, reduction in mortalities, and an attendant increase in life expectancies.[6] This "rising Africa" with an enlarging working and consuming population and a potential driving force for global economic growth is expecting an increase in persons with disability (PWD) in the years to come.[2,5,6] Along with the increase in longevity, increasing incidence of road traffic accidents, conflicts, and chronic noncommunicable diseases (NCDs) contribute to the increase in disability in the continent.[2,5,9,10] Africa needs updated disaggregated disability statistics to drive political decision making, and objective planning of rehabilitation services and disability support programs.[11]

As in any low- and middle-income country, most African nations have incomplete disability statistics limited to impairment-based prevalence data that largely focus on the most visible forms of limitations of functions.[9,11] The World Report on Disability prevalence estimates for moderate and moderate to severe disability in Africa are 3.1% and 15.3%, respectively.[9] Infectious diseases are still the leading cause of disability in most African countries, although intentional and unintentional injuries and NCDs prevalence are on the increase.[5,6,10] In most African countries, disability data segregated by age, gender, and impairment types are scarce.[9,10] Information on the contribution of contextual factors to limitations of activities and participations, and physical environment suitability map for PWD with various impairments are exceptions in Africa.[9,10] Biopsychosocial conceptualization and analysis of disability under International Classification of Functioning (ICF) framework should be reconsidered in the local contexts and demands to operationalize disability measures for comprehensive disability data collection.[12,13]

Africa needs now, more than ever, working policy frameworks, commitments, and collaborations to fulfill the civic, social, cultural, economic, and political rights of PWD. As already pointed out, the African region, having limited resources, is undergoing demographic transition in unstable sociopolitical environment that potentially increases the complexity and magnitude of disability.[5,6,10] Currently, several nations in Africa have national disability policy and laws to realize and facilitate different rights of an ever-increasing community of PWD.[10] However, disability promotion, prevention, and rehabilitation services are poorly harmonized, integrated, and monitored.[10] Implementation of disability policies and strategies in the continent has thus been suboptimal.[10] Intersectoral coordination and collaboration with local and international nongovernmental organizations (NGOs) are required in disability and development-related activities.[10] Participation of the continent's PWD and disability people organizations (DPOs) in planning and implementation of all disability-related activities will enhance their self-determination and mitigation of barriers to rehabilitation.[10]

Community-based rehabilitation (CBR) programs in Africa should be supported with resources and good governance practices. Founded on the philosophy of primary health care (PHC), CBR focuses on the provision of essential rehabilitation and support services for PWD and their families using locally available resources and full local community participation.[8,14–16] However, its implementation did not get beyond strategic adoption, fractured services, and pilot programs in most African countries.[10] In Africa, most CBR programs are concentrated in major cities and poorly linked with health-related rehabilitation (HRR) services.[8,10] They are inaccessible to most PWD who live in rural areas of Africa.[8,10] Available CBR programs largely focus on economic, education, and social activities, and health components, including assistive devices, are covered by few of the CBR.[10] Furthermore, CBR have raised programmatic and pragmatic concerns that need to be appropriately redressed.[8,14,17,18] Inadequate funding, infrastructure, and trained CBR providers and lack of integrated evaluation and implementation strategies for its activities continued to be the major obstacles for quality CBR services.[8,17,18] Poor political commitment and insufficient participation of DPOs and PWD contribute to CBR's suboptimal acceptance and sustainability.[8,17,18] CBR in Africa should be strengthened to develop a robust and evolving theoretic framework for academic analysis, and to have clear leadership structure and infrastructure conducive for training and research.[18]

In Africa, where health expenditure is stagnant at an average of nearly 5% of gross domestic product, rehabilitation service delivery strategies should be explored for their feasibility and sustainability.[1,5,19] In the Global North service models and treatment philosophy, comprehensive rehabilitation services rely on interlinked infrastructures, skilled rehabilitation professionals, and efficient program management.[19] Postacute rehabilitation services are the continuum of care provided at different distinct and free-standing inpatient and outpatient rehabilitation centers.[19] Multitudes of skilled rehabilitation service providers are involved, including physician specialists, rehabilitation nurses, different therapists, technicians, social workers, and case managers.[19] Inevitably, Africa, with suboptimal general health coverage and governance practices, will stagger in implementing the Global North rehabilitation service model. Currently, average composite indexes for general service availability and readiness in Africa are 59% and 62%, respectively.[20] Locally responsive delivery strategies are needed for accessible and equitable multidisciplinary rehabilitation services in Africa.[5,20]

Barriers to comprehensive and quality multidisciplinary rehabilitation services in Africa are suggested in various studies.[1,3,4,9,20–22] Multidisciplinary rehabilitation workforces are inadequate and poorly coordinated into teams, resulting in fragmented and ineffective CBR and HRR services.[4,21,23,24] In most African countries, teamwork spirit and cross-disciplinary learning culture are not meaningfully cultivated to deliver a coordinated continuum of rehabilitation care.[24] Interprofessional misunderstanding and practice barriers resulted in duplication of roles, incoordination of efforts, and compartmentalization of rehabilitation skills in community CBR workers, allied health rehabilitation professionals, and rehabilitation physicians.[24] Available skilled rehabilitation professionals are concentrated in the major cities and large hospitals and are inaccessible to most people with rehabilitation needs in rural areas and community settings.[10,22,24] Highly skilled rehabilitation service providers are less motivated financially and carrier-wise to practice in the CBR programs in the continent.[22–24]

In Africa, clients with disability and rehabilitation needs have poor access to general health care and rehabilitation services with an unacceptably high risk for secondary health problems and worse health outcomes.[9,21,22] Available rehabilitation services in

Africa are often unaffordable to PWD, who are usually unemployed and economically drained.[20–22] Health and rehabilitation service infrastructures are not uncommonly physically inaccessible and led by staff with poor understanding of disability.[9,22] Health care providers and related stakeholders lack awareness to multidimensional needs of PWD and have inadequate knowledge and skills to provide rehabilitation services.[24] Moreover, rehabilitation care in Africa is misconceived and underfunded and left for charity and religious NGOs.[8,10,20,21] Health care systems are poorly linked to community CBR programs and have poor involvement in rehabilitation services and information collection.[1,10,25] The management and governance problems have perpetuated the health inequality and poor health outcomes for PWD and contributed to inadequate multidisciplinary rehabilitation workforce development efforts in the continent.[21,26]

In most African countries, rehabilitation professional training programs are few, fragmented, and poorly designed for facilitation of interprofessional learning and collaboration.[21,23,25,27] Available rehabilitation workforces are poorly defined and monitored to quantify and direct rehabilitation human resource development.[21,25] Most African rehabilitation service provider training programs focus on community workers and allied health professionals.[25,27] They are ineffective in integrating rehabilitation agenda in regular health professional training curricula and development of diverse multidisciplinary rehabilitation workforces.[25,27] Getting practicing physiatrists or physiatrist training programs is not easy in Africa.[3,21,25,26] Rehabilitation physician specialists are relevant for quality of rehabilitation services, rehabilitation workforce training, CBR program implementation, and the continent's contribution to the global disability and rehabilitation literature.[3,10,28,29] Disability research in Africa is inadequate and requires capacity building and partnership with local rehabilitation professionals.[1,30,31]

There is no need to emphasize the health, economic, and social benefits of investment on rehabilitation in Africa.[20,21] Africa should abide by its commitments and development of partnership to alleviate the challenges for accessible, equitable, and client-centered comprehensive rehabilitation services.[9,32,33] Multisectoral and multistakeholder coordination and strategic partnerships for rehabilitation services and governance are suboptimal in sub-Saharan Africa (SSA).[1,25,29] Nonexistent or inadequate funding for rehabilitation services and scarcities of rehabilitation facilities and equipment are clearly observable in SSA.[1,4] Poor integration of rehabilitation in the existing health care systems impacts the quality of rehabilitation practices in the continent.[1,20] Working and flexible partnerships and collaborations are key for successful implementation of rehabilitation interventions and practices.[34–36]

REHABILITATION SERVICES IN AFRICA: LESSONS LEARNED

Although not uniform and consistent, global cooperation for rehabilitation in Africa has brought noticeable changes over the last few decades. International partnerships for disability research have laid the groundwork for future opportunities by setting standard practice framework for research collaboration.[34,35,37,38] The continent has seen innovative approaches for rehabilitation service delivery that positively changed the disparities PWD in Africa are facing.[39,40] International collaborative efforts for physiatric training programs have been encouraging.[41] Improved rehabilitation leadership and interdisciplinary education have enhanced rehabilitation services and hopes of people with rehabilitation needs in few countries in Africa.[24,36]

North-south partnerships for disability research in Africa have increasingly exemplified a participatory approach and regional collaborations in the continent. EquitAble ("Enabling universal and equitable access to healthcare for vulnerable people in resource poor settings in Africa") is a multicountry and multidisciplinary research project funded by the European Commission Seventh Research Framework Programme to identity factors influencing access to health care for vulnerable groups in 4 African countries.[37] Researchers and institutions from Europe and 4 host African countries had maintained a balanced and close working relationship at all project stages.[37] They met early in the project to extensively discuss local contextual factors that helped in determining research problems and development of concept papers specific to each host country.[37] Since these early meetings, involvement of PWD (as researchers) and DPOs (as consultants) from the local communities has been maintained till completion of data collection.[37] Moreover, frequent meetings during the project offered opportunities for cultural transfer, mutual learning, and realization of effective intraregional research collaborations.[37] Similarly, Aldersey and Wenda[38] capitalized on not only the Participatory Action Research approach that ensures social validity and reflexivity of research but also the need to communicate research results to communities and to do periodic impact evaluation of research.

In a few African countries, innovative approaches have helped to empower PWD and bridge the information gap on availability of disability services. A project funded by Google Impact Challenge-disability grant developed smart phone application software that tracks and maps the availability of disability services, including assistive technology (AT) in southern Africa.[39] The software created in consultation with local stakeholders (DPOs, PWD, AT suppliers, and intermediaries) and international experts was an offline user-friendly freely downloadable application that can be used by people with various types of disabilities.[39] In a pilot testing of the software in Botswana, it was received well by all stakeholders and allowed quick and efficient access to AT products by customers.[39] It was reported that the cost of AT has decreased (shorter supply chain), and sense of empowerment in PWD has increased because of the software.[39] Wheelchair users trained as peer trainers in Kenya and Malawi have empowered PWD as service providers and reduced the sense of social isolation in participants of the project.[40] Also, the peer trainers (wheelchair users) trained on various issues of mobility impairments (health, wheelchair skills, and PWD rights) have positively influenced the knowledge, skills, and quality of life of their peers (**Fig. 1**).[40]

The International Rehabilitation Forum (IRF) pioneering local physiatric training in SSA launched parallel online physical medicine and rehabilitation (PMR) fellowship programs in Ghana and Ethiopia in September 2018.[41] The IRF is a 15-year-old consortium of universities and individuals around the world dedicated to building medical rehabilitation where it is not available by advocacy, policy consultation, leadership training, and assisting local projects for sustainable PMR training programs and rehabilitation services.[41] Consistent with its philosophy, IRF developed a balanced and working relationship with dedicated local partners in Ghana (Ghana College of Family Medicine) and Ethiopia (St. Paul's Hospital Millennium Medical College).[42] In consultation with IRF and other partners, host institutions designed locally responsive and reflexive 2-year physiatry fellowship curricula.[42] The fellowship is primarily online based and has been ongoing through a secure electronic communication platform of the University of Michigan.[42] In the next 4 years, the fellowship will build core teaching staff in the countries to sustain it locally.[42] This first local SSA PMR fellowship, which thus far is too early to tell about their impacts and outcomes, illustrates viable approaches and platforms for collaborations that need to be explored by academic institutions and professional societies around the world (**Fig. 2**).

Efforts of the Uganda Society for Disabled Children (USDC) in strengthening HRR services at PHC settings in Uganda demonstrate some of the positive impacts of partnerships and linkages between CBR and HRR services.[24] As a Ugandan registered

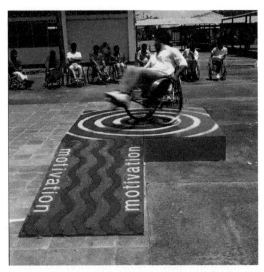

Fig. 1. Peer wheelchair training session. Demonstration of wheelchair skills on ramp walkway. Motivation Peer Training programme in Managua, Nicaragua, teaching new wheelchair users the skills to become more mobile and independent © Motivation. (*From* Norris L. 'Introducing: Motivation's revised peer training package'. Available at: https://www.motivation.org.uk/blog/introducing-mpt; with permission.)

NGO, USDC implemented CBR among children with disabilities and their families in several districts of the country.[24] In an attempt to extend its services, USDC started supporting service infrastructures and specific disability in-service training of rehabilitation specialists within the PHC settings.[24] In so doing, the USDC was able to reach more children with disabilities and succeeded in getting HRR issues on the district's agenda with increased funding priority and inclusion of rehabilitation package in PHC outreach programs.[24] On a broader scale, interprofessional education and collaborative practice (IECP) could allow joint participatory planning, task-sharing, and willingness to change in partnership.[24] In line with the principles of IECP, Faculty of Community and Health Sciences at the University of the Western Cape, South Africa implemented an interdisciplinary community-based practice module to facilitate open communication, mutual understanding, knowledge and skills exchanges, and acquisition of teamwork skills among students of various health disciplines.[36] It is clear that strong political framework, enabling legislation, and shared health governance models

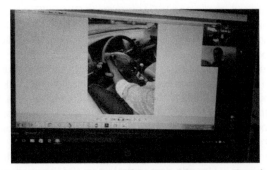

Fig. 2. Online physiatry fellowship. Case presentation session on roles of orthotics and assistive devices on community integration of people with disability.

are key determinants for realization of interprofessional education and teamwork spirit among the currently fragmented rehabilitation service providers and stakeholders.[36]

The aforementioned partnership and practice models of rehabilitation services and research in the continent are just a few, and their selection is by no means based on stringent outcome and impact evaluation criteria. However, envisaging a better future for PWD in Africa, they give an overview of past experiences of rehabilitation practices in the continent to relevant stakeholders around the world.

THE FUTURE OF REHABILITATION SERVICES IN AFRICA

Rehabilitation consists of a package of interventions that optimize functioning and minimize disability of persons with many disabling health conditions at various service settings.[1] For rehabilitation in the health care setups, access to elements of rehabilitative, assistive, and palliative care should be assured and integrated with the usual health services at all levels of the health care system.[1,20] In any country, accessible, affordable, and quality rehabilitation in an integrated people-centered health services framework is instrumental for achievement of the targets in sustainable development goal-three (SDG-3) and effective implementation of other health strategies, such as mental health action plan, global cooperation on assistive technology, and global strategy and action plan on aging and health.[1] Countries in Africa should mobilize resources for comprehensive rehabilitation services as per the recommendations stipulated in Rehabilitation 2030: A Call For Action and Rehabilitation in Health System strategic plan documents contextually adapted to their specific needs and priorities.[1,20]

Creating strong political support, appropriate policies, and good governance for rehabilitation at subnational, national, and regional levels is critical for efficient service delivery and positive rehabilitation outcomes.[1,43] Well thought-out strategic policy frameworks will bring about good leadership and governance of rehabilitation practices, including HRR and CBR services, AT delivery, disability advocacy, rehabilitation workforce training, research, and financing.[1,43] In Africa, rehabilitation policy development, implementation, and monitoring processes need to be participatory and transparent, and reflexive of the dynamic contextual factors that potentially influence the specific policy frameworks of each country.[43] Participation of PWD and DPOs in policy processes is essential to improve rehabilitation program responsiveness, efficiency, effectiveness, and sustainability, and to strengthen service-user empowerment and satisfaction.[43] National rehabilitation policy should explicitly promote access to services and PWD to support equitable and accessible rehabilitation services.[43] Strong intersectoral coordination and multistakeholder collaboration should be led by coherent policy mandates for each governmental ministry and department regarding the provision of various rehabilitation services and activities.[43] Governance and leadership of rehabilitation programs should be clearly institutionalized, aligning with preexisting governmental health care models of individual African countries.[43] Rehabilitation leadership and governance also involve effective oversight, coalition building, provision of appropriate regulations and incentives, and attention to service design.[43]

In all African countries, availability of disability and rehabilitation data should be strengthened to support political momentum, decision making by policymakers, equitable allocation of resources, rehabilitation and assistive strategies, governance, and evaluation.[1,43] Disaggregated disability statistics help in justifying the need for rehabilitation.[1] Disability information derived from population surveys and administrative data that rely on performance of individuals with disabilities in their environment (bottom-up approach) is more accurate than epidemiologic studies of disabling conditions (top-down approach) in estimating the need for rehabilitation.[1] Countries are encouraged to regularly update disability data in population surveys and health care facilities using the bottom-up approach and ICF framework.[1,12] System level disability and rehabilitation data collection should be included in the existing health information system of health care institutions.[1] Collection of rehabilitation data at health care facilities is possible when the health care facilities provide rehabilitation and stewardship of non–health rehabilitation services.[1] Also, building the research capacity and expanding the availability of robust evidences for economic, social, and health benefits of rehabilitation helps in making the case for rehabilitation investment.[1]

A comprehensive rehabilitation service delivery model for equitable access to quality services, including assistive devices, for all the population should be adopted by all countries in Africa.[1] Strengthening of the existing health service infrastructures might be required to effectively integrate rehabilitation at all levels of the health systems.[20,36] Moreover, CBR programs in Africa demand strong bidirectional referral linkage with HRR.[20,24] Intersectoral links among governmental ministries and departments Involved in rehabilitation should be strengthened to effectively and efficiently meet the needs of PWD.[1] Financing rehabilitation through appropriate mechanisms is relevant in most African countries.[1] Insurance coverage for rehabilitation is a feasible option that may be advocated in Africa. The road accident fund (RAF) in South Africa, for example, is a social security safety net that solicits compulsory social insurance coverage to all users of South African roads.[44] The RAF covers costs of rehabilitation care and community integration of motor vehicle accident survivors in South Africa.[44] Third-party payers for rehabilitation, such as national health insurance, are critical in reducing barriers to care when available, in addition to providing incentives for medical facilities to establish rehabilitation programs.

Each country in Africa should have a strong multidisciplinary rehabilitation workforce suitable for their contexts.[1] Appraisal of the stocks and profiles of available rehabilitation workforces is a proxy estimate for rehabilitation need and assists in planning customized and relevant training programs.[1,22,25–27,29] In Africa, where there are dire shortages of rehabilitation specialists, rehabilitation training programs that facilitate IECP might be justified.[24,36] IECP cultivates the techniques and culture of teamwork among rehabilitation professionals.[24,36] Integrated rehabilitation training programs create platforms for interactions and exchange of knowledge and skills among allied health professional trainees. Physiatry training programs in Africa, at least for a few years to come, should equip graduate fellows with leadership qualities and required levels of skills to provide various aspects of rehabilitation. Having a few cadres of such physiatrists in each African country might improve the current status of multidisciplinary rehabilitation services in SSA. These physiatrists may spearhead and organize multidisciplinary rehabilitation services in remote and most urban areas of Africa. Physiatrists play key roles in leading and monitoring of IECP-guided integrated rehabilitation training programs of allied health professionals. Promoting rehabilitation concepts and CBR elements across all health workforce education and training curricula improve awareness and development of rehabilitation practices in Africa.[1] Rehabilitation professionals in Africa should engage in teaching and monitoring of CBR workers on health aspects of rehabilitation.[36]

Strategic partnerships of stakeholders at various levels are required for better rehabilitation practices in SSA.[1,25,29] Often, concerns and problems of rehabilitation practices in Africa need to be addressed based on long-term partnerships and commitments among stakeholders and engagement of local community.[34] Long-term successful partnerships usually come from involvement of higher officials and prominent personalities at institutional levels.[34,35] Consultation of existing local partners early in the process of identifying priorities and implementation planning is essential for sustainability of collaborative rehabilitation programs.[34,35,37] Periodic evaluation of the rehabilitation programs serves to improve program implementation and mutual trust among involved parties.[34,35,38] Moreover, cooperation and partnerships on rehabilitation programs should consider the multidisciplinary and multidimensional nature of rehabilitation care.[34,35] The social, economic, health, and political facets, and the attendant need for multiple professionals in rehabilitation, are part of the equation in alleviating the continent's unmet needs for comprehensive evidence-based rehabilitation services.[1,45] As experience tell us, mobile applications platforms, telerehabilitation, and 3-dimensional printing will have a bigger role in rehabilitation in Africa.[39,41]

SUMMARY

Currently, Africa has huge unmet needs for rehabilitation services, which are expected to widen with the trend for an increase in disabling conditions and longevity in the continent. Despite policies and legislations, most African countries have not yet realized accessible and equitable comprehensive continuum of rehabilitation care. There should be considerations for policy and service model adjustments and strengthening of collaborations at all levels to positively impact barriers to rehabilitation services and assistive devices. Rehabilitation services should be integrated into the health care systems and form supportive relationship with CBR programs in the continent. The place of technologies and innovative approaches in hastening rehabilitation services in the continent should be explored.

REFERENCES

1. World Health Organization. The need to scale up rehabilitation. Background briefing paper for the meeting Rehabilitation 2030: a call for action. Geneva (Switzerland): WHO; 2017. Available at: http://www.who.int/disabilities/care/rehab-2030/en. Accessed September 10, 2018.
2. Vos T, Flaxman AD, Naghavi M, et al. Years lived with disability (YLDs) for 1160 sequelae of 289 diseases and injuries 1990-2010: a systematic analysis for the Global Burden of Disease Study 2010. Lancet 2012;39:2163–96.
3. Haig AJ, Im J, Adewole A, et al. The practice of physical medicine and rehabilitation in sub-Saharan Africa and Antarctica: a white paper or a black mark? Disabil Rehabil 2009;31(13):1031–7.
4. Gupta N, Castillo-Laborde C, Landry MD. Health-related rehabilitation services: assessing the global supply of and need for human resources. BMC Health Serv Res 2011;11:276. Available at: https://doi.org/10.1186/1472-6963-11-276. Accessed September 12, 2018.
5. World Health Organization. Atlas of African health statistics 2018: universal health coverage and the sustainable development goals in the WHO African region. Brazzaville (Congo): WHO Regional Office for Africa; 2018. Licence: CC BY-NC-SA 3.0 IGO.
6. World Health Organization. The health of the people: what works. The African regional health report. Brazzaville (Congo): WHO Regional Office for Africa; 2014. Available at: https://afro.who.int/publications/african-regional-health-report-2014-health-people-what-works. Accessed September 19, 2018.
7. World Health Organization. WHO global disability action plan 2014–2021. Better health for all people with disability. Geneva (Switzerland): WHO;

2015. Available at: http://www.aho.afro.who.int/sites/default/files/publications/921/AFROStatistical_Factsheet.pdf?ua=1. Accessed August 29, 2018.

8. Kuilers P, Sabuni LP. Community-based rehabilitation and disability-inclusive development: on a winding path to an uncertain destination. In: Grech S, Soldatic K, editors. Disability in the global south, international perspectives on social policy, administration, and practice: the critical. Cham (Switzerland): Springer International Publishing Company, Inc; 2016. p. 453–67.

9. World Health Organization and World Bank. World report on disability. Geneva (Switzerland): WHO; 2011. Available at: http://www.whqlibdoc.who.int/publications/2011/9789240685215_eng.pdf. Accessed September 20, 2018.

10. World Health Organization. Disability and rehabilitation status: review of disability issues and rehabilitation services in 29 African countries. Geneva (Switzerland): WHO; 2004.

11. Eide AH, Loeb M. Counting disabled people: historical perspectives and the challenges of disability statistics. In: Grech S, Soldatic K, editors. Disability in the global south, international perspectives on social policy, administration, and practice: the critical handbook. Cham (Switzerland): Springer International Publishing Company, Inc; 2016. p. 51–68.

12. World Health Organization. International classification of functioning, disability and health. Geneva (Switzerland): WHO; 2001. Available at: http://whqlibdoc.who.int/publications/2011/9789240685215_eng.pdf. Accessed September 29, 2018.

13. Goodley D, Swartz L. The place of disability. In: Grech S, Soldatic K, editors. Disability in the global south, international perspectives on social policy, administration, and practice: the critical handbook. Cham (Switzerland): Springer International Publishing Company, Inc; 2016. p. 69–84.

14. Lemmi V, Gibson L, Blanchet K, et al. Community based rehabilitation for people with disabilities in low- and middle-income countries: a systematic review, 3ie Systematic Review 18. London: International Initiative for Impact Evaluation; 2015 (3ie).

15. World Health Organization. Community-based rehabilitation: CBR guidelines 2010a. Geneva (Switzerland): WHO; 2010. Available at: http://www.who.int/disabilities/10/guidelines/en/. Accessed July 19, 2018.

16. International Labour Organization, United Nations Educational, Scientific and Cultural Organization, World Health Organization. CBR: A strategy for rehabilitation, equalization of opportunities, poverty reduction and social inclusion of people with disabilities. Joint Position Paper 2004. Geneva, Switzerland: WHO; 2004. Available at: http://www.who.int/disabilities/publications/10/en/index.html. Accessed August 10, 2018.

17. Saurabh S, Prateek S, Jegadeesh R. Exploring the scope of community-based rehabilitation in ensuring the holistic development of differently-abled people. Afr Health Sci 2015;15(1):278–9.

18. World Health Organization. International consultation to review community-based rehabilitation (CBR). Geneva (Switzerland): WHO; 2003. Available at: http://www.whqlibdoc.who.int/hq/2003/who_dar_03.2.pdf. Accessed August 20, 2018.

19. Keith RA, Aronow HU. Comprehensive rehabilitation: themes, models, and issues. In: Zaretsky HH, Richter EF III, Eisenberg MG, editors. Medical aspects of disability: a handbook for the rehabilitation professional. 3rd edition. New York: Springer Publishing Company, Inc; 2005. p. 3–29.

20. World Health Organization. Rehabilitation in health systems. Geneva (Switzerland): WHO; 2017. Licence: CC BY-NC-SA 3.0 IGO. Available at: http://www.who.int/disabilities/rehabilitation_health_systems/en/. Accessed Jan 12, 2018.
21. Jesus TS, Landry MD, Dussault G, et al. Human resources for health (and rehabilitation): six rehab-workforce challenges for the century. Hum Resour Health 2017;15(1):8.
22. Bright T, Wallace S, Kuper H. A systematic review of access to rehabilitation for people with disabilities in low-and middle-income countries. Int J Environ Res Public Health 2018;15:2165.
23. Wylie K, McAllister L, Davidson B, et al. Rehabilitation in sub-Saharan Africa. A workforce profile of speech and language therapists. Afr J Disabil 2016;5:13.
24. Nganwa AB, Batesaki B, Mallya JA. The link between health-related rehabilitation and CBR. In: Musoke G, Geiser P, editors. Linking CBR, disability and rehabilitation. Bangalore (India): 10 Africa Network; 2013. p. 60–70.
25. Agho AO, John EB. Occupational therapy and physiotherapy education and workforce in Anglophone sub-Saharan Africa countries. Hum Resour Health 2017;15:37.
26. Hasheem M, Malcolm M, Eilish M. The human resources challenge to community based rehabilitation: the need for a scientific, systematic and coordinated global response. Disability, CBR and Inclusive Development Journal 2012;23:4.
27. Cornielje H, Majisi J, Locoro V. Capacity building in CBR: learning to do CBR. In: Musoke G, Geiser P, editors. Linking 10, disability and rehabilitation. Bangalore, India: 10 Africa Network; 2013. p. 53–7.
28. Tinney MJ, Chiodo A, Wiredu E. Medical rehabilitation in Ghana. Disabil Rehabil 2007;29:921–7.
29. Dalton SC. The current crisis in human resources for health in Africa: the time to adjust our focus is now. Trans R Soc Trop Med Hyg 2014;108:526–7.
30. Cleaver S, Nixon S. A scoping review of 10 years of published literature on community-based rehabilitation. Disabil Rehabil 2014;36:1385–94.
31. Jesus TS. Systematic reviews and clinical trials in rehabilitation: comprehensive analyses of publication trends. Arch Phys Med Rehabil 2016;97:1853–62.e2.
32. United Nations. Convention on the rights of persons with disabilities. New York: UN; 2006. Available at: http://www.un.org/disabilities/convention/conventionfull.shtml. Accessed September 20, 2018.
33. United Nations. Sustainable development goals: sustainable development knowledge platform. New York: UN; 2015. Available at: https://sustainabledevelopment.un.org/sdgs. Accessed August 14, 2018.
34. Walker RJ, Campbell JA, Egede LE. Effective strategies for global health research, training and clinical care: a narrative review. Glob J Health Sci 2015; 7(2):119–39.
35. Fisher KR, Shang X, Xie J. Global south-north partnerships: intercultural methodologies in disability research. In: Grech S, Soldatic K, editors. Disability in the global south, international perspectives on social policy, administration, and practice: the critical handbook. Cham (Switzerland): Springer International Publishing Company, Inc; 2016. p. 567–82.
36. Fefoame GO, Walugembe J, Mpofu R. Building partnerships and alliance in CBR. In: Musoke G, Geiser P, editors. Linking CBR, disability and rehabilitation. Bangalore (India): 10 Africa Network; 2013. p. 37–50.
37. MacLachlan M, Amin M, Mji G, et al. Learning from doing the EquitAble project: content, context, process, and impact of a multi-country research project on

vulnerable populations in Africa. Afr J Disabil 2014;3(2). https://doi.org/10.4102/ajod.v3i2.89.

38. Aldersey H, Wenda DA. Partnerships for disability research in Africa: lessons learned in Kinshasa, Democratic Republic of the Congo. Disabil Global S 2015;2(3):777–93.

39. Visagie SJ, Matter R, Kayange GM, et al. Lessons from the pilot of a mobile application to map assistive technology suppliers in Africa. Afr J Disabil 2018;7(0):a422.

40. Norris LK. Motivation peer training–bridging the gap for people with mobility disabilities. Afr J Disabil 2017;6(0):a350.

41. International Rehabilitation Forum. International rehabilitation forum: medical rehabilitation for the world. Available at: http://www.rehabforum.org/index.html. Accessed November 2, 2018.

42. St. Paul's Hospital Millennium Medical College, International Rehabilitation Forum. Physical medicine and rehabilitation: fellowship curriculum. Addis Ababa (Ethiopia): St. Paul's Hospital Millennium Medical College; 2017. p. 2–8.

43. Joanne M, Malcolrn M, Brynne G, et al. Promoting good policy for leadership and governance of health related rehabilitation: a realist synthesis. Global Health 2016. https://doi.org/10.1186/s12992-016-0182-8.

44. Road Accident Fund. RAF rehabilitation services. Available at: https://www.raf.co.za/Product-and-Services/Pages/Rehabilitation.aspx. Accessed November 26, 2018.

45. World Health Organization. World Conference on Social Determinants of Health: meeting report. Rio De Janeiro, Brazil: WHO. 2011. Available at: https://www.who.int/sdhconference/resources/wcsdh_report/en/. Accessed November 12, 2018.

Development of Rehabilitation in China

Jianan Li, MD[a],*, Leonard S.W. Li, MBBS, FRCP, FAFRM(RACP), FHKAM(Medicine)[b,c]

KEYWORDS

- Disability • China • Rehabilitation • Future development

KEY POINTS

- The population with disability in China comprises 85 million permanently disabled persons, more than 200 million persons with disabilities from chronic diseases, and more than 240 million elderly persons.
- Delivery of rehabilitation services in China includes rehabilitation in general hospitals, specialized rehabilitation hospitals, community-based rehabilitation, and home-based rehabilitation.
- Rehabilitation personnel are lacking in Mainland China. The number of required rehabilitation physicians, therapists, and nurses is estimated to be 60,000, 150,000, and 60,000, respectively in the coming 10 years.
- Investment in rehabilitation services in both public and private sectors will increase dramatically in the near future through the influence of Chinese Government policy.

EPIDEMIOLOGY OF DISABILITY

Accurate data on epidemiology of disability in China is not available owing to the lack of a national registry of disability as well as an evolving definition and concept of disability during the past 10 years.

In China, a disabled person is defined as one with permanent or long-lasting disabilities with significant influence on independence of life. The World Health Organization global disability action plan 2014 to 2021 declared that disability is universal. Everybody is likely to experience disability directly or to have a family member who experiences difficulties in functioning at some point in his or her life, particularly as they grow older. "Disability" is an umbrella term for impairments, activity limitations, and participation restrictions, denoting the negative aspects of the interaction between an individual (with a health condition) and that individual's contextual (environmental and

Disclosure Statement: The authors have nothing to disclose.
[a] Medical Rehabilitation Center, Nanjing Medical University, Nanjing, China; [b] Neurological Rehabilitation Centre, Virtus Medical Center, 11th Floor, Virtus Medical Tower, 122 Queen's Road Central, Central, Hong Kong SAR, China; [c] Department of Medicine, University of Hong Kong, Hong Kong SAR, China
* Corresponding author.
E-mail address: lijianan@carm.org.cn

Phys Med Rehabil Clin N Am 30 (2019) 769–773
https://doi.org/10.1016/j.pmr.2019.07.010

personal) factors. Therefore, the population with disability in China should include 85 million permanently disabled persons, more than 200 million persons with disabilities from chronic diseases, and more than 240 million elderly persons (ie, aged 60 years or older) (**Fig. 1**) who have difficulty leading an independent life. China has a total population of 1.39 billion. Although there may be some overlap among the aforementioned population, the data reflect the overall status of disability in China.

In the adult population, the prevalent major chronic diseases are hypertension (25.2%) and diabetes (9.7%). Cancer, cerebral vascular disease, coronary artery disease, and respiratory disease are the major cause of death and disabilities (**Table 1**). **Table 1** also shows a significant increase in heart disease and a decrease in respiratory disease in rural areas. Chronic diseases are responsible for 79.5% of deaths in urban and 85.3% in suburban areas.

The percentage of persons with low physical activity is 35.9% and the proportion undertaking regular exercise amounts to only 18.7%. Most persons with low physical activity have various disabilities, including poor mobility from paralysis and weakness, low cardiopulmonary function and aerobic capacity, fatigue, depression and anxiety, and limited independence in activities of daily living. Social recognition of this situation is increasing significantly in the general population as well as policy makers in government. Therefore, medical rehabilitation has been promoted dramatically since 2008, when the Wenchuan earthquake resulted in 100,000 dead or missing persons.

DEVELOPMENT OF REHABILITATION SERVICES

The availability of rehabilitation services has tripled during the past 10 years (**Fig. 2**). Current models of rehabilitation services delivery in China include: departments of rehabilitation in general hospitals, specialized rehabilitation hospitals, community-based rehabilitation, and home-based rehabilitation. There are 2 types of hospitals, government and private. During the past 10 years, the number of private rehabilitation hospitals (**Fig. 3**) and the capacity of inpatient beds (**Fig. 4**) have increased significantly.

Manpower in Medical Rehabilitation

A national survey in 2009 found that there were 16,000 physicians, 14,000 therapists, and 12,000 nurses in medical rehabilitation. The latest data in 2018 reported 38,260 physicians and 15,514 nurses in rehabilitation hospitals. It is estimated that there approximately 40,000 therapists in practice. The projected need in 10 years for rehabilitation physicians, therapists, and nurses is estimated to rise to approximately

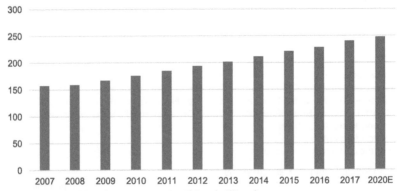

Fig. 1. Population older than 60 years in China (millions).

Table 1
Changes in mortality in urban and rural populations in China from 2005 to 2017 (deaths expressed as 1 per 100,000)

	2005				2017			
	Urban		Rural		Urban		Rural	
	Deaths	Rate (%)	Deaths	Rate (%)	Deaths	Rate (%)	Deaths	Rate (%)
Cancer	164.35	26.44	105.99	20.08	160.72	26.11	156.70	23.07
Brain disease	128.23	20.63	111.74	21.17	126.58	20.65	157.48	23.18
Heart disease	136.61	21.98	62.13	11.77	141.61	23.00	154.40	22.73
Respiratory disease	73.36	11.80	123.79	23.45	67.20	10.92	78.57	11.57

60,000, 150,000, and 60,000, respectively. As of 2018, there were 225 schools for therapist training, which is projected to increase to about 300 in 2025. Currently, there are approximately 10,1000 graduates from these schools per year, and the numbers continue to increase significantly. The goal of most of the programs will be to train general therapists. More therapist training programs meeting international standards are planned in the disciplines of physical therapy, occupational therapy, speech pathology, and prosthetics and orthotics. In addition, in the near future, it is expected that subspecialty programs in pediatric rehabilitation, geriatric rehabilitation, manual therapy, and traditional Chinese therapy, as well as therapy with specialty competencies, will be developed.

FUTURE DEVELOPMENT

In 2009, the Chinese government announced the national health care strategy, comprising the 3 major key elements of prevention, treatment, and rehabilitation, followed by a series of national documents "Standard of department of rehabilitation and guideline for management in general hospitals (2011)," "Standard of rehabilitation hospitals (2012)," "Principles of early rehabilitation intervention for 9 common diseases (2013)," "Guidance on medical rehabilitation for the 12th Five-Year Plan period (2015)," "Promotion of industry in smart assistive devices and robotics (2016)," and "Standard of medical rehabilitation centers and nursing homes (2017)."

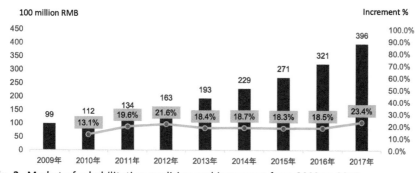

Fig. 2. Market of rehabilitation medicine and increment from 2009 to 2017.

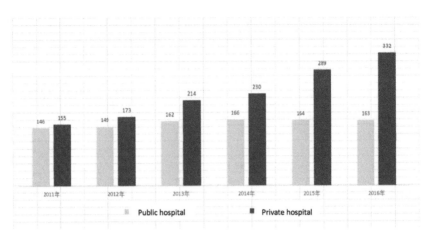

Fig. 3. Trend of rehabilitation hospitals (public versus private) from 2011 to 2016.

The most important national document is "Outline of Healthy China 2030". The 6 key principles related to rehabilitation medicine are

A. Integrating health as a priority strategic policy in all government departments to ensure health in every aspect and over the whole lifespan for all citizens.
B. Early diagnosis, early treatment, and early rehabilitation to facilitate rehabilitation in all clinical specialties, especially orthopedics, neurology and neurosurgery, cardiology, respiratory medicine, endocrinology, oncology, pediatrics, geriatrics, intensive care unit, chest surgery, gynecology and obstetrics, ophthalmology, ear/nose/throat, psychology, mental disease, pain management, material addiction, and subhealth conditions.
C. Complete service chain in health care from treatment to rehabilitation and long-term care. Establishment of extended services is encouraged, including rehabilitation hospitals, long-term care facilities, and nursing facilities, as well as community rehabilitation services.
D. Traditional Chinese medicine to help in acute medical care and to be a core element in rehabilitation and a key measure for prevention.
E. To promote the health industry as a pillar industry, especially with regard to smart assistive devices, rehab robotics, prosthesis and orthosis, virtual reality, new materials, wearable devices, meta-data collection and analysis, and remote medicine.
F. Cross-border integration: emphasis on integration of sports with medicine, senior service with medicine, and engineering with medicine.

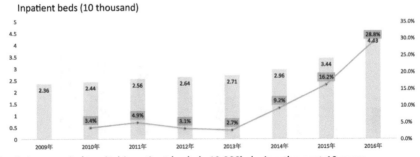

Fig. 4. Increase in hospital inpatient beds (×10,000) during the past 10 years.

Based on these principles, social investment in rehabilitation services is increasing dramatically. Almost all provinces have initiated projects such as "Healthy town," "Town for rehabilitation and senior care," and "Cluster of rehabilitation hospital, nurse home, and sports and recreation center."

A new government department, the State Medical Security Bureau, was established in 2018. This is the first government body to integrate insurance management, and will significantly influence the future direction of medical services and long-term care. The Bureau has responsibilities for basic medical insurance for urban and rural residents, maternity insurance, managing prices of drugs and medical services, and humanitarian medical support. These responsibilities had been managed by multiple government bodies in the past, including the State Health and Family Planning Commission, the Ministry of Human Resources and Social Security, the State Development and Reform Commission, and the Ministry of Civil Affairs. The State Medical Security Bureau has been set up as an organ directly under the State Council.

Recently, insurance policies have changed from Item-Related Grading to Diagnostic-Related Grading and Function-Related Grading. Two national research projects, "Functional evaluation and grading for senior population based on ICF" and "Functional evaluation and grading for long-term care," are under way and will be completed by the end of 2019. These changes may play an important role in guiding insurance policy for medical and long-term care. Clinical implementation of ICF (International Classification of Functioning, Disability and Health) is also being initiated in hospitals and other medical facilities.

Prolotherapy for Musculoskeletal Pain and Disability in Low- and Middle-Income Countries

David Rabago, MD[a],*, Kenneth Dean Reeves, MD[b], Mary P. Doherty, RTR[c], Maelu Fleck, BS[d]

KEYWORDS

- Prolotherapy • Osteoarthritis • Tendinopathy • Chronic pain
- Low- and middle-income countries • Regenerative therapy

KEY POINTS

- Chronic musculoskeletal pain and disability reduce the quality and quantity of life worldwide, with a disproportionately high impact in low- and middle-income countries.
- Traditional, complementary, and integrative medicine may have much to offer in the prevention and treatment of chronic musculoskeletal pain and disability.
- Prolotherapy is an injection-based complementary therapy that addresses causes of pain and disability at the tissue level, supported by high-quality evidence for osteoarthritis, tendinopathy, and low back pain.
- Prolotherapy is a straightforward office-based procedure that relies on common, inexpensive materials, and does not require refrigeration, making it an attractive treatment option in low- and middle-income countries.
- Although not typically part of conventional medical training, not-for-profit organizations are teaching clinicians and treating patients with prolotherapy in low- and middle-income countries through service-learning projects.

Disclosure: None of the authors have a financial relationship with a commercial company that has a direct financial interest in subject matter or materials discussed in this article. Organizations discussed are nonprofit (501c3). D. Rabago is immediate past president and member of the board of directors of the Hackett Hemwall Patterson Foundation; K.D. Reeves is a member of the board of directors of the American Association of Orthopaedic Medicine; neither are paid for these efforts. M.P. Doherty and M. Fleck are paid vice president and executive director of the Hackett Hemwall Patterson Foundation and American Association of Orthopaedic Medicine, respectively.
[a] UW Department of Family Medicine and Community Health, University of Wisconsin School of Medicine and Public Health, 1100 Delaplaine Court, Madison, WI 53715, USA; [b] Private Practice, Physical Medicine and Rehabilitation, 4740 El Monte Street, Roeland Park, KS 66205, USA; [c] Hackett Hemwall Patterson Foundation, 2532 Baldwin Street, Madison, WI 53713, USA; [d] American Association of Orthopaedic Medicine, 3700 East Quebec Street, 100-236, Denver, CO 80207-1639, USA
* Corresponding author.
E-mail address: david.rabago@fammed.wisc.edu

Phys Med Rehabil Clin N Am 30 (2019) 775–786
https://doi.org/10.1016/j.pmr.2019.07.003
1047-9651/19/© 2019 Elsevier Inc. All rights reserved.

GLOBAL IMPACT OF BACK PAIN, OSTEOARTHRITIS, AND TENDINOPATHY

Musculoskeletal (MSK) health problems are major contributors to the global burden of disease as assessed by the metric "years lived with disease" (YLD). They cause 21.3% of the total burden as measured by YLD, second only to mental and behavioral problems,[1,2] and are a worldwide threat to healthy aging. Some MSK conditions cause disproportionate impact; low back pain (LBP) is the leading specific cause of YLD-defined disability, "other MSK disorders," which include heterogeneous conditions including chronic tendon- and ligament-related pain, ranked sixth, and hip and knee osteoarthritis (OA), ranked 11th.[3,4]

Low- and middle-income countries, where MSK conditions are the third greatest threat and cause of death and disability, experience a disproportionate burden.[1,2] Characteristics predisposing to MSK problems and common in higher-income countries include an aging demographic and increasing obesity. Associations resulting in disproportionate MSK burden in low- and middle-income countries include rapid population growth, the high-intensity physical nature of much subsistence work, and the general poor access to health promotion and treatment services.[5]

Government and aid organizations have historically focused less on MSK and more on life-threatening conditions, such as communicable diseases, and building the overall health care capacity. Content experts have called for more attention, indeed a "paradigm shift," among global agencies to address the large and growing burden of disability caused by MSK conditions. They have suggested large-scale policy change and local efforts at the level of international health agencies, such as the World Health Organization (WHO) and national health agencies, and have advocated for the use of core principles of local ownership, local decision-making, community and stakeholder engagement, integration of services into the larger policy and structures, and avoidance of current unimodal approaches. Particularly relevant to this report is the call for collaboration with international organizations and local stakeholders in the pursuit of community-based treatment efforts.[5]

Although such calls to action are clear and evidence based, they may ignore a group of potential impactful therapies that have not gained a broad recognition. Often missing from discussions about treatment of MSK conditions on a global scale is the category of traditional, complementary, and integrative medicine (TCIM). October 2018 marked the 40th anniversary of the WHO Alma Ata Declaration, a document which established health as a human right and placed the development of primary health care at the center of global health priorities.[6] It also identified TCIM as having a place in health care systems. Primary care "relies, at local and referral levels, on health workers, including physicians, nurses, midwives, auxiliaries, and community workers as applicable, as well as traditional practitioners as needed, suitably trained socially and technically to work as a health team and to respond to the expressed health needs of the community."[6] This declaration was among the first major policy statements to both acknowledge TCIM in primary care and suggest its potential to make a positive impact on health.

WHO defines TCIM medicine as a "broad set of health care practices that are not part of that country's own tradition and are not integrated into the dominant health system."[7] Numerous well-known, evidence-based TCIM therapies, including meditation, acupuncture, yoga, tai chi, massage, and other movement and body techniques, as well as prolotherapy, may offer solutions to some MSK chronic pain and disability in low- and middle-income countries.

PROLOTHERAPY
Definition and History

Prolotherapy is an emerging injection-based TCIM therapy for chronic MSK conditions used by both primary care and MSK specialty clinicians.[8] Less well-known than some TCIM MSK therapies, prolotherapy was developed in the United States in the early and middle twentieth century, and remains largely outside conventional medicine. Prolotherapy is most often taught using peer learning, and in conference, workshop, and formal continuing medical education settings. However, the evidence base supporting prolotherapy is growing, and includes effectiveness and efficacy studies for treatment of high-burden conditions of OA and LBP, and in ligament and tendon disorders owing to overuse. Prolotherapy is unique in its capacity to deliver active therapy to a variety of local tissue and pain generators, both within and around joint spaces in a single treatment session. Treatment materials are inexpensive and require no cold chain; the injection protocols, although operator dependent, are straightforward to learn using palpation guidance.[9-11] Prolotherapy may therefore have application to the growing burden of MSK pain and disability in low- and middle-income countries. In this article, we define prolotherapy, provide an review of evidence, and describe the efforts of 2 nonprofit organizations to introduce prolotherapy to low- and middle-income countries through humanitarian service-learning projects.

Developed in the early twentieth century, the first peer-reviewed report about prolotherapy appeared in 1937.[12] George Hackett, MD, a general surgeon in the United States, later formalized injection techniques based on clinical experience and research. Believing tissue proliferation to be an essential aspect of the effects of the injections, he named the procedure: "To the treatment of proliferating new cells, I have applied the name prolotherapy."[13] Because the purported effects of prolotherapy include revitalization and reorganization of degenerative tissue, it has also been categorized by some content experts as a "regenerative" injection therapy.[14] Practitioners have refined the injection protocols using consensus-based efforts to provide guidelines and clinical practice.[9]

Treatment commonly consists of several injection sessions conducted every 4 to 8 weeks over several months. Hypertonic dextrose is the most commonly used injectant. During a treatment session, dextrose is injected at sites of tender ligament and tendon attachments, and also in adjacent joint spaces.[15] It is hypothesized that the solutions that are injected cause local irritation, with subsequent inflammation and anabolic tissue healing, which improves joint stability, biomechanics, function, and, ultimately, decreases pain.

Mechanism of Action

A tissue-level pain-control mechanism is hypothesized but has not been well elucidated; however, it is likely multifactorial, involving effects at multiple tissue types and planes, and associated with both the physical injection procedure and the biological effects of the injectant. Mechanistic studies of dextrose prolotherapy suggest a noninflammatory proliferant effect,[16-18] potential clinical effects via brief stimulation of the inflammatory cascade,[19] chondrogenesis,[20] and a clinical analgesic effect with or without hypertonic levels of dextrose.[21,22]

Conditions for Which Prolotherapy Is Evidence Based

The first systematic review of prolotherapy for all indications for MSK found 42 published reports from 1937 to 2005.[8] Thirty-six were case reports or case series and reported positive findings for patients with a wide variety of chronic, painful MSK conditions refractory to then-current best care; the strength of methodology varied among these studies. Most of the participants assessed were treated for LBP; other conditions included knee and finger OA, shoulder dislocation, neck strain, costochondritis, lateral epicondylosis, and fibromyalgia. These pragmatic studies assessed prolotherapy in clinical settings and provided the platform from which to perform more formal studies. Prolotherapy has primarily been subjected to a descriptive review inclusive of all randomized clinical trials and included 15 such studies. The rate of publication of high-quality clinical trials is accelerating.[23] Here, we review the major studies most relevant for 3 sets of conditions, OA, tendinopathy, and LBP, which are of particular relevance to low- and middle-income countries.

Osteoarthritis

Of all indications for which prolotherapy is used, clinical trial data best support its use for OA. Early studies by Reeves and Hassanein[24,25] assessing intra-articular dextrose injections for knee and finger OA reported efficacy compared with control injections, and suggested the need for more rigorous study. Two groups conducted more rigorous trials of prolotherapy for knee OA. Using the validated Western Ontario McMaster University Osteoarthritis Index (WOMAC) (0–100-point scale), they documented improvement after prolotherapy of more than 12 points, which is the minimal clinically important difference on the WOMAC scale for knee OA.[26,27]

Rabago and colleagues[15] conducted an open-label pilot study of prolotherapy and established methodological elements, effect size, and overall feasibility for a randomized controlled trial (RCT). Participants reported 15.9 points of improvement on the overall WOMAC scores. Shortly thereafter, Dumais and colleagues[28] corroborated these findings in a crossover study in which participants who received physical therapy and prolotherapy were compared with patients receiving physical therapy alone. At 16 weeks, prolotherapy was added to the physical therapy group; and the change on the aggregate WOMAC scale attributed to prolotherapy alone was 11.9 points.

Using injection protocols from their pilot study, Rabago and colleagues[21] compared prolotherapy with at-home exercise and blinded saline injection in a 3-arm RCT. Prolotherapy participants reported statistically and clinically relevant score improvement compared with both control groups at 9, 24, and 52 weeks, culminating in a 15.3-point improvement on the WOMAC assessment: nearly twice that of the controls. These are the most robust data favoring prolotherapy, and suggest that prolotherapy, performed by a trained operator, results in safe, substantial, and sustained improvement on knee-specific quality of life indicators. Three systematic reviews, 2 with meta-analyses, found that prolotherapy resulted in significant, clinically important improvement for knee OA without adverse events concurred with these findings.[29–31] A subsequent open-label study followed participants to an average of 2.5 years postenrollment and reported continued improvement to an average of 20.9 points on the WOMAC scale.[32] Of these participants, 82% improved compared with their baseline status; however, 18% worsened, consistent with the natural history of knee OA. No study has identified baseline predictive markers of success with prolotherapy.

Tendinopathies

There is also evidence that prolotherapy is successful in several chronic, painful conditions caused by tendon overuse. The purported mechanism of prolotherapy is well matched to the current understanding of tendinopathy caused by tendon overuse, because it is primarily a noninflammatory, degenerative condition. We provide a description of selected studies for tendinopathies of particular relevance to low- and middle-income countries: lateral epicondylosis (LE), Achilles tendon, and rotator cuff tendinopathies. Other MSK conditions not reviewed here, but which are also supported by high-quality data, include hip adductor and patellar tendinopathy, plantar fasciopathy, and temporomandibular joint dysfunction.[33,34]

Lateral epicondylosis or tennis elbow Two pilot-level RCTs suggest that prolotherapy is efficacious for LE. In a 2-arm study comparing prolotherapy with blinded saline injections, Scarpone and colleagues[35] assessed 20 adults (10 per group) with severe LE refractory to standard care and who were considering surgery. Participants who were treated with prolotherapy reported, on a 0 to 10 point visual analog scale (VAS), significantly decreased scores over 16 weeks of 4.6 points, whereas controls reported decreased scores of 1.0 point. Participants who received prolotherapy also showed significantly improved isometric strength compared with controls, and improved grip strength compared with baseline status. These clinical improvements in prolotherapy subjects were maintained at 52 weeks. These data were corroborated by Rabago and colleagues[36] in a pilot study using the Patient-rated Tennis Elbow Evaluation, a validated measure of primary outcome. Both studies suggest efficacy but are limited by small sample size. Data from both studies were used to establish methods for an ongoing, more definitive study.[37]

Achilles tendinopathy Maxwell and colleagues[38] conducted a case series (N = 36) to assess whether prolotherapy, injected under ultrasound guidance, decreases pain and changes ultrasound-based parameters of tendon character. At 52 weeks, participants reported improvement in VAS-assessed pain severity by 88%, 84%, and 78% during rest, "usual" activity, and sport, respectively. Tendon thickness decreased significantly; however, other ultrasound-based criteria were not correlated with self-reported outcomes. Prolotherapy has been assessed in a high-quality RCT comparing prolotherapy, physiotherapy, and combined care. Participants reported earlier response, and the study reported improved cost-effectiveness, when physiotherapy and prolotherapy were combined, compared with either treatment alone.[39]

Rotator cuff tendinopathy Bertrand and colleagues[40] assessed use of prolotherapy for rotator cuff tendinopathy in a 3-arm blinded RCT. Patients received prolotherapy, blinded injection, or superficial blinded injections at 0, 1, and 2 months. The primary outcome was improvement in shoulder pain greater than or equal to 2.8 points on 0 to 10 using the VAS. The percentage of participants receiving prolotherapy meeting this criterion was statistically greater than in the controls who received the superficial lidocaine injection (59% vs 27%), but not in the group who received the lidocaine injection (59% vs 37%). These findings suggest that the study may have been underpowered or that the deep lidocaine injections had a treatment effect above that of placebo. The findings were incorporated into a systematic review and compared with several different injection therapies for symptomatic rotator cuff syndrome. Network meta-analysis showed that prolotherapy was superior to other injection therapies in pain reduction at long-term follow-up.[41]

Chronic low back pain
Four RCTs have assessed prolotherapy for nonsurgical nonspecific LBP; 3 used phenol-glycerine-glucose (P2G) as the injectant[42–44]; the fourth and most rigorous trial used dextrose.[45] Each RCT used a protocol involving injections to the ligamentous attachments of the L4-S1 spinous processes, sacrum, and ilium. Although many outcome measures varied across the studies, the percentage of participants reporting over 50% improvement in pain and disability scores at 6 months was a common assessment.

In the methodologically strongest RCT, participants were randomized to 1 of 4 groups: dextrose and physical therapy, dextrose and "normal activity," saline injections and physical therapy, or saline injections and normal activity.[45] At 12 months, participants in all groups reported reduced pain (by 26%–44%) and disability (by 30%–44%) scores; the percentage of participants who reached at least a 50% pain reduction ranged from 36% and 46% across the groups. Change in outcome scores favored the dextrose groups, but not by statistically significant margins. Most (55%) reported that improvement in pain and disability had been worth the effort of undergoing the study interventions. Whereas the study was reported as negative, subtler interpretation is reasonable. Two factors likely served to limit detection of a therapeutic effect favoring the active arm. First, sham injection procedures contain several therapeutic components, including needle stick, pressure/volume tissue-level changes, and acute injury from needle stick on bone with initiation of blood-based irritation and inflammatory healing cascade.[46] Each would minimize the difference between control and active injection groups. Second, the study was likely under powered given the use of such an active control.

Direct sensorineural effects of dextrose are suggested by the results of a novel RCT assessing dextrose administered as an epidural injection. Maniquis-Smigel and colleagues[22] compared serial blinded 5% dextrose injections with saline injectant in 35 participants with chronic LBP and buttock or leg pain. A statistically significant analgesic effect was seen in those who received dextrose in comparison with those who received normal saline injections, which lasted from 15 minutes to 48 hours (P<.05); this effect endured with repeated injection in a longer-term follow-up study.[47] The speed of analgesia onset after an epidural injection suggests a potential direct effect of dextrose at the level of peripheral nerves.

Interpretation of LBP prolotherapy trials is challenging; methodological questions have been raised.[48] A systematic review[49] found insufficient evidence to recommend prolotherapy for nonspecific LBP; however, while early clinical trial data offer generally promising results, more rigorous, sufficiently powered trials are needed. Studies assessing prolotherapy in patients with more narrowly focused diagnoses of LBP have been done in an effort to determine the underlying pathology most responsive to prolotherapy. Cusi and colleagues[50] assessed 25 participants with sacroiliac joint dysfunction refractory to 6 months or more of physical therapy, and noted improvements in pain and disability scores at follow-up after 26 months. Khan and colleagues[51] assessed 37 adults with coccydynia refractory to other care, and also noted a reduction in pain scores from 8.5 to 2.5 points at 2 months. Miller and colleagues[52] assessed prolotherapy as an intradiscal injection for leg pain in participants who had an imaging-confirmed moderate-to-severe degenerative disc disease, and who had not responded to either physical therapy or 2 fluoroscopically guided epidural corticosteroid injections. After an average of 3.5 sessions of biweekly, fluoroscopically guided intradiscal injections with 25% dextrose, 43% showed a significant, sustained treatment response. Although these studies of prolotherapy for focused causes of LBP were uncontrolled, they suggest the effectiveness and the need for further research to assess the use of prolotherapy for specific causes of LBP.

Contraindications/Side Effects and Adverse Events

Prolotherapy seems safe when practiced by a trained clinician. Injections should be performed using universal precautions. Contraindications, side effects, and adverse events have been reviewed.[23] There are few absolute contraindications to prolotherapy, and include skin or joint infection, rheumatological flare, allergy to injectant, and treatment with immunosuppressive medications. Relative contraindications include gouty arthritis flare, acute fracture, bleeding disorders, and use of anticoagulants. After prolotherapy treatment, patients may report acute injection-related discomfort and tissue "fullness." Pain occurs in approximately 10% of patients within the first 72 hours postinjection.[21] Additional injection-related procedural risks include lightheadedness, allergic reaction, infection, or nerve injury.

PROLOTHERAPY AND SERVICE-LEARNING ORGANIZATIONS

Although prolotherapy is not generally taught in conventional medical education centers, organizations with a focus on so-called regenerative injection therapies offer conference and workshop instruction, and limited training worldwide (**Table 1**). At least 2 of these organizations also do service-learning work, with some projects in low- and middle-income countries; these include the American Association of Orthopaedic Medicine (AAOM) and the Hackett Hemwall Patterson Foundation (HHPF). Their work exemplifies a means of dissemination of the teaching and practice of prolotherapy, while delivering care to underserved populations.[53,54] Each of these organizations has developed a curriculum, teaching style, and practice standards, which include didactic and workshop training in conference settings in the United States and intensive, hands-on clinical practice experiences in low- and middle-income countries; the HHPF has developed a formal set of procedural guidelines to structure these experiences.[9]

The AAOM was founded in 1983 by physicians from the United States and Canada to advance nonsurgical Orthopaedic medicine. The roots of the HHPF extend to 1969, when founders established an annual service trip to Honduras to provide prolotherapy to the underserved. While both organizations have grown to include other activities, each provides prolotherapy for chronic MSK pain through their service-learning work. The organizations and their service-learning trips share several characteristics. Each organization is a 501c3 not-for-profit entity and conducts medically oriented trips in Latin America that integrate service and learning. Each organization conducts hands-on prolotherapy training as part of a larger service project. Licensed physicians enroll in the fee-based experience, which is eligible for continuing medical education credit in the United States. The learning experience includes on-site lectures and demonstration, and mentored hands-on experience in clinics established for the project that provide free care to local patients. Both groups also train local clinicians in prolotherapy at no cost. Locations include 3 cities in Honduras (La Ceiba, Tela, and Olanchito), 2 in Mexico (Guadalajara and Cancun), and 1 in Peru (Lima). Both groups work with other regional centers. Local partners vary and include community groups, churches, the Honduran Red Cross, local physician groups, and university departments (see **Table 1**). At each site, representatives of AAOM or HHPF work with local partners to establish temporary clinics, inform patients of care options provided free of charge or at nominal cost, obtain consent for prolotherapy care, complete relevant history and examination, and obtain basic demographic information. Patients are treated on a first-come, first-served basis; local interpreters are available on-site to enable a real-time communication between the patients and the treating clinicians. Patients are examined to establish whether prolotherapy is appropriate for them; if so, prolotherapy is explained, and interested patients complete an informed consent for the procedure. Patients are treated using standards of medical professionalism, hygiene, and procedural safety that mirror those of the United States. Existing prolotherapy teaching materials are used; the HHPF also uses standardized teaching materials for procedural approaches to each joint/area that have been developed using a

Table 1
Characteristics of prolotherapy service-learning trips of 2 North American medical organizations

Organization	Clinic Location	Inception Date	Local Partner Organization	Duration of Service-Learning Project (wk)	Average Number of Patients Undergoing Prolotherapy	Number of Visiting Trainees	Number of Local Trainees
HHPF	La Ceiba, Honduras	1969	Cruz Roja Hondureña (Red Cross)	2	650	4–7	1–2
	Tela, Honduras	1988	Sala Evangelica Church	2	600	4–7	1–2
	Olanchito, Honduras	2004	Community leader and Sociedad de Agricultores y Ganaderos de Olanchito (SAGO)	2	550	4–7	1–2
	Guadalajara, Mexico	2006	Palabra de Vida Church and local physician	1	575	17–18	2–3
AAOM	Cancun, Mexico	2007	Local mayor, community government, and local Department of Family Medicine	1	600	12–16	6
	Lima, Peru	2011	Clinica Internacional del Peru, local PM&R clinics, and local physician	1	450	8–12	6
	Guadalajara, Mexico	2013	Universidad de Guadalajara, Hospital Civil de Guadalajara, and local physician	1	600	12–16	6

Abbreviations: AAOM, American Association of Orthopaedic Medicine; HHPF, Hackett Hemwall Patterson Foundation; PM&R, physical medicine and rehabilitation.

Table 2	
Medical organizations providing didactic and hands-on prolotherapy instruction	
Australia	
Australian Association of Musculoskeletal Medicine	https://aamm.org.au/courses-conference/
Asia	
Hong Kong Institute of Musculoskeletal Medicine	http://www.hkimm.hk/
Taiwan Association of Prolotherapy and Regenerative Medicine	http://www.taprm.org/
Europe	
European School of Prolotherapy	proloterapia.it/en/
North America	
American Association of Orthopaedic Medicine	aaomed.org/
The American Osteopathic Association of Prolotherapy Regenerative Medicine	prolotherapycollege.org/
Canadian Association of Orthopaedic Medicine	Caom.ca
Hackett Hemwall Patterson Foundation	hhpfoundation.org/
South America	
Latin American Association of Orthopaedic Medicine	www.laomed.org

All URLs accessed March 18, 2019; the table presents a sample of prolotherapy learning opportunities worldwide.

consensus model by organization members who are experts in prolotherapy techniques.[9]

The service-learning projects offered by both groups have a successful track record of patient care safety and, anecdotally, positive impact on health; each organization safely treats over 1000 patients annually and trains dozens of physicians. Anecdotally, patients express satisfaction with care; many return each year for treatment of the same or other MSK conditions. Side effects and adverse events are rare and do not seem to exceed those in developed countries. In addition to these 2 leading organizations, other medical groups have formed. On occasion, students and teachers from these 2 "parent" organizations have gone on to found their own teaching groups; one can now learn prolotherapy worldwide (**Table 2**). Such growth suggests an increasing interest among clinicians and patients in prolotherapy, and points the way to efforts that can scale up this care worldwide. A short-term goal common to all such organizations is to build in mechanisms to systematically assess project-specific patient and community outcomes to better understand the effect of such efforts. Longer-term efforts should include improved local community and other stakeholder involvement, and integration of training efforts into formal medical education and policy considerations.

ACKNOWLEDGMENTS

Portions of the section "Conditions for Which Prolotherapy is Evidence Based" are adapted with permission from D. Rakel (*Integrative Medicine, 4th Ed.*, 1047–1053. Philadelphia: Elsevier; 2018). The following physicians contributed information about prolotherapy teaching outside of North America: Regina Sit, Asia; Michael Yelland and Margi Taylor, Australia; Steven Cavallino, Europe; Francois Louw and Adrian Gretton, Canada; Gaston Topol, South America.

REFERENCES

1. Murray CJ, Vos T, Lozano R. Disability-adjusted life years (DALYs) for 291 diseases and injuries in 21 regions, 1990–2010: a systematic analysis for the Global Burden of Disease Study. Lancet 2013;380:2197–223.
2. Vos T, Flaxman AD, Naghavi M. Years lived with disability (YLDs) for 1160 sequelae of 289 diseases and injuries 1990–2010: a systematic analysis for the Global Burden of Disease Study 2010. Lancet 2013;380:2163–96.
3. Smith E, Hoy DG, Cross M, et al. The global burden of other musculoskeletal disorders: estimates from the Global Burden of Disease 2010 study. Ann Rheum Dis 2014;73:1462–9.
4. Cross M, Smith E, Hoy D, et al. The global burden of hip and knee osteoarthritis: estimates from the global burden of disease 2010 study. Ann Rheum Dis 2014;73:1323–30.
5. Hoy D, Geere JA, Davatchi F, et al. A time for action: opportunities for preventing the growing burden and disability from musculoskeletal conditions in low- and middle-income countries. Best Pract Res Clin Rheumatol 2014;28:377–93.
6. WHO. Declaration of Alma-Ata: International Conference on Primary Health Care, vol. 32. Geneva (Switzerland): WHO Chron; 1978. p. 428–30. PMID: 11643481.
7. WHO. Essential medicines and health products information portal: a World Health Organization resource 2002. Available at: http://apps.who.int/medicinedocs/en/d/Js2297e/4.1.html#Js2297e.4.1. Accessed March 6, 2019.
8. Rabago D, Best T, Beamsly M, et al. A systematic review of prolotherapy for chronic musculoskeletal pain. Clin J Sport Med 2005;15(5):376–80.
9. Hackett Hemwall Patterson Foundation. Basic prolotherapy study guide. Madison (WI): Hackett Hemwall Patterson Foundation; 2017. Available at: http://hhpfoundation.org/.
10. Ravin T, Cantieri M, Pasquarello G. Principles of prolotherapy. Denver (CO): American Academy of Musculoskeletal Medicine; 2012.
11. Baumgartner JJ. Regenerative injections: the art of healing complete injection manual. 7th edition. Waite Park (MN): Rejuvmedical; 2018. Available at: http://regenerative-md.com/.
12. Schultz L. A treatment for subluxation of the temporomandibular joint. JAMA 1937;109(13):1032–5.
13. Hackett GS, Hemwall GA, Montgomery GA. Ligament and tendon relaxation treated by prolotherapy. 5th edition. Madison (WI): Hackett Hemwall Patterson Foundation; 1993. Available at: http://hhpfoundation.org/.
14. DeChellis DM, Cortazzo MH. Regenerative medicine in the field of pain medicine: prolotherapy, platelet-rich plasma, and stem cell therapy—theory and evidence. Tech Reg Anesth Pain Manag 2011;15(2):74–80.
15. Rabago D, Zgierska A, Fortney L, et al. Hypertonic dextrose injections (prolotherapy) for knee osteoarthritis: results of a single-arm uncontrolled study with 1-year follow-up. J Altern Complement Med 2012;18:408–14.
16. Oh S, Ettema AM, Zhao C, et al. Dextrose-induced subsynovial connective tissue fibrosis in the rabbit carpal tunnel: a potential model to study carpal tunnel syndrome? Hand (N Y) 2008;3:34–40.
17. Yoshii Y, Zhao C, Schmelzer JD, et al. Effects of hypertonic dextrose injections in the rabbit carpal tunnel. J Orthop Res 2011;29:1022–7.
18. Yoshii Y, Zhao C, Schmelzer JD, et al. Effects of multiple injections of hypertonic dextrose in the rabbit carpal tunnel: a potential model of carpal tunnel syndrome development. Hand (N Y) 2014;4:52–7.

19. Jensen KT, Rabago D, Best TM, et al. Early inflammatory response of knee liga-
    ments to prolotherapy in a rat model. J Orthop Res 2008;26(6):816–23.
20. Topol GA, Podesta L, Reeves KD, et al. The chondrogenic effect of intra-articular
    hypertonic-dextrose (prolotherapy) in severe knee osteoarthritis. PM R 2016;8:
    1072–82.
21. Rabago D, Patterson JJ, Mundt M, et al. Dextrose prolotherapy for knee osteoar-
    thritis: a randomized controlled trial. Ann Fam Med 2013;11(3):229–37.
22. Maniquis-Smigel L, Reeves KD, Rosen JH, et al. Short term analgesic effect of
    caudal 5% dextrose epidural injection for chronic low back pain. A randomized
    controlled trial. Anesth Pain Med 2017;7(1).
23. Reeves KD, Sit RW, Rabago DP. Dextrose prolotherapy: a narrative review of
    basic science, clinical research, and best treatment recommendations. Phys
    Med Rehabil Clin N Am 2016;27(4):783–823.
24. Reeves KD, Hassanein K. Randomized, prospective, placebo-controlled double-
    blind study of dextrose prolotherapy for osteoarthritic thumb and finger (DIP, PIP,
    and trapeziometacarpal) joints: evidence of clinical efficacy. J Altern Comple-
    ment Med 2000;6(4):311–20.
25. Reeves KD, Hassanein K. Randomized prospective double-blind placebo-
    controlled study of dextrose prolotherapy for knee osteoarthritis with or without
    ACL laxity. Altern Ther Health Med 2000;6(2):77–80.
26. Ehrich E, Davies G, Watson D, et al. Minimal perceptible clinical improvement
    with the Western Ontario and McMaster Universities osteoarthritis index question-
    naire and global assessments in patients with osteoarthritis. J Rheumatol 2000;
    27(11):2635–41.
27. Tubach F, Wells G, Ravaud P, et al. Minimal clinically important difference, low
    disease activity state, and patient acceptable symptom state: methodological is-
    sues. J Rheumatol 2005;32(10):2025–9.
28. Dumais R, Benoit C, Dumais A, et al. Effect of regenerative injection therapy on
    function and pain in patients with knee osteoarthritis: a randomized crossover
    study. Pain Med 2012;13:990–9.
29. Sit RWS, Chung VCH, Reeves KD, et al. Hypertonic dextrose injections (prolother-
    apy) in the treatment of symptomatic knee osteoarthritis: a systematic review and
    meta-analysis. Sci Rep 2016;6:25247.
30. Hassan F, Trebinjac S, Murrell D, et al. The effectiveness of prolotherapy in treat-
    ing knee osteoarthritis in adults; a systematic review. Br Med Bull 2017;122:
    91–108.
31. Hung CY, Hsiao MY, Chang KV, et al. Comparative effectiveness of dextrose pro-
    lotherapy versus control injections and exercise in the management of osteoar-
    thritis pain: a systematic review and meta-analysis. J Pain Res 2016;9:847–57.
32. Rabago D, Mundt M, Zgierska A, et al. Hypertonic dextrose injection (prolother-
    apy) for knee osteoarthritis: long term outcomes. Complement Ther Med 2015;
    23(3):388–95.
33. Louw F, Reeves KD, Lam SKH, et al. Treatment of temporomandibular dysfunction
    with hypertonic dextrose injection (prolotherapy): a randomized controlled trial
    with long-term partial crossover. Mayo Clin Proc 2019;94(5):820–32.
34. Reeves KD, Sit RWS, Rabago D. A narrative review of basic science and clinical
    research, and best treatment recommendations. Phys Med Rehabil Clin N Am
    2016;27:783–823.
35. Scarpone M, Rabago D, Zgierska A, et al. The efficacy of prolotherapy for lateral
    epicondylosis: a pilot study. Clin J Sport Med 2008;18(3):248–54.

36. Rabago D, Lee KS, Ryan M, et al. Hypertonic dextrose and morrhuate sodium injections (prolotherapy) for lateral epicondylosis (tennis elbow): results of a single-blind, pilot-level randomized controlled trial. Am J Phys Med Rehabil 2013;92(7):587–96.

37. Yelland M, Rabago D, Bisset L, et al. Randomised clinical trial of prolotherapy injections and an exercise program used singly and in combination for refractory tennis elbow. Queensland (Australia): Griffith University; 2014. Available at: https://wwwanzctrorgau/Trial/Registration/TrialReviewaspx?ACTRN=12612000993897.

38. Maxwell NJ, Ryan MB, Taunton JE, et al. Sonographically guided intratendinous injection of hyperosmolar dextrose to treat chronic tendinosis of the Achilles tendon: a pilot study. AJR Am J Roentgenol 2007;189:W215–20.

39. Yelland MJ, Sweeting KR, Lyftogt JA, et al. Prolotherapy injections and eccentric loading exercises for painful Achilles tendinosis: a randomised trial. Br J Sports Med 2011;45:421–8.

40. Bertrand H, Reeves KD, Bennett CJ, et al. Dextrose prolotherapy versus control injections in painful rotator cuff tendinopathy. Arch Phys Med Rehabil 2016;97(1):17–25.

41. Lin MI, Chiang CF, Wu CH, et al. Comparative Effectiveness of Injection Therapies in Rotator Cuff Tendinopathy: A Systematic Review, Pairwise and Network Meta-analysis of Randomized Controlled Trials. Arch Phys Med Rehabil 2018;100:336–49.

42. Ongley MJ, Klein RG, Dorman TA, et al. A new approach to the treatment of chronic low back pain. Lancet 1987;2:143–6.

43. Klein RG, Eek BC, DeLong WB, et al. A randomized double-blind trial of dextrose-glycerine-phenol injections for chronic, low back pain. J Spinal Disord 1993;6(1):23–33.

44. Dechow E, Davies RK, Carr AJ, et al. A randomized, double-blind, placebo-controlled trial of sclerosing injections in patients with chronic low back pain. Rheumatology 1999;38:1255–9.

45. Yelland M, Glasziou P, Bogduk N, et al. Prolotherapy injections, saline injections, and exercises for chronic low back pain: a randomized trial. Spine 2004;29(1):9–16.

46. Rabago D, Wilson JJ, Zgierska A. Letter to the editor; platelet-rich plasma for treatment of Achilles tendinopathy. JAMA 2010;303:1696–7.

47. Maniquis-Smigel L, Reeves KD, Rosen HJ, et al. Analgesic effect and potential cumulative benefit from caudal epidural D5W in consecutive participants with chronic low-back and buttock/leg pain. J Altern Complement Med 2018. https://doi.org/10.1089/acm.2018.0085.

48. Reeves KD, Klein RG, DeLong WB. Letter to the editor. Spine 2004;29(16):1839–40.

49. Yelland MJ, Del Mar C, Pirozo S, et al. Prolotherapy injections for chronic low back pain: a systematic review. Spine 2004;29:2126–33.

50. Cusi M, Saunders J, Hungerford B, et al. The use of prolotherapy in the sacro-iliac joint. Br J Sports Med 2008;44:100–4.

51. Khan SA, Kumar A, Varshney MK, et al. Dextrose prolotherapy for recalcitrant coccygodynia. J Orthop Surg 2008;16:27–9.

52. Miller MR, Mathews RS, Reeves KD. Treatment of painful advanced internal lumbar disc derangement with intradiscal injection of hypertonic dextrose. Pain Physician 2006;9:115–21.

53. Hackett Hemwall Patterson Foundation. 2019. Available at: http://hhpfoundation.org/. Accessed August 06, 2019.

54. American Association of Orthopaedic Medicine. 2019. Available at: https://www.aaomed.org/default.aspx. Accessed August 06, 2019.

Rehabilitation in Nepal

Raju Dhakal, MBBS, MD[a],*, Christine C. Groves, MD[a,b,1]

KEYWORDS

- Rehabilitation • Nepal • Low- and middle-income countries • Disability

KEY POINTS

- Rehabilitation services in Nepal are limited, but the government has recently adopted a 10-year action plan to address rehabilitation needs nationwide.
- Rehabilitation education and training are necessary to provide and retain adequate multidisciplinary rehabilitation providers for current and future needs in Nepal.
- Implementation of evidence-based recommendations to improve the quality of rehabilitation services and access to rehabilitation is critical to maximize individual and community well-being.

INTRODUCTION

Nepal is a landlocked, mountainous country situated in South Asia between China and India (**Fig. 1**), with an estimated population of 29.9 million and life expectancy at birth of 70 years.[1,2] The World Bank categorizes Nepal as a low-income country, with a gross national income per capita of $790 and more than 25% of the population living below the poverty line.[2]

The term rehabilitation is broadly defined as "a set of interventions designed to optimize functioning and reduce disability in individuals with health conditions in interaction with their environment."[3] Thus, rehabilitation extends to many different specialties and sectors of society. For the purpose of this article, therefore, we specifically focus on medical rehabilitation, including physical medicine and rehabilitation physicians; therapy, including physiotherapy, occupational therapy, and speech and language conditions; and assistive devices.

In addition, rehabilitation is needed and used by a wide variety of individuals, ranging from those with acute injuries who recover fully to those with chronic medical conditions and long-term disabilities. This article specifically focuses on rehabilitation

Disclosure Statement: The authors have nothing to disclose.
[a] Physical Medicine and Rehabilitation, Spinal Injury Rehabilitation Centre, Post box no 13815, Sanga 011-660847, Nepal; [b] Department of Physical Medicine and Rehabilitation, Indiana University School of Medicine, Indianapolis, IN, USA
[1] Present address: 4204 Ponderosa Boulevard, Indianapolis, IN 46250.
* Corresponding author.
E-mail address: dr.rajupmr@gmail.com

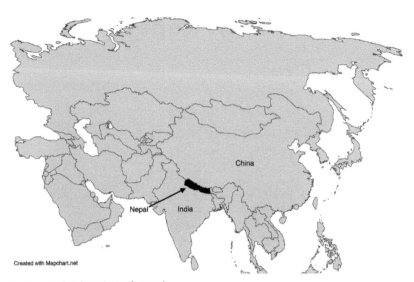

Created with Mapchart.net

Fig. 1. Geographic location of Nepal.

that addresses physical impairments and the resultant hindrances that affect an individual's full and effective participation in society, as defined by the Convention on the Rights of Persons with Disabilities (CRPD).[4] Notably, we do not include impairments, disabilities, and rehabilitation services related to mental and hearing/vision impairments, which are themselves enormous fields beyond the scope of this article.

The objectives of this article are to:

- Summarize known data pertaining to the current need for rehabilitation in Nepal.
- Review the present state of rehabilitation services in Nepal.
- Recommend next steps to further develop rehabilitation services appropriate to the needs and context of Nepal.

NEED FOR REHABILITATION

There have been no comprehensive rehabilitation needs assessments completed in Nepal. However, given that more than 90% of the causes of the world's burden of disease may benefit from rehabilitation services, the potential needs are significant.[5] Here, we present global and national data addressing both disability and health conditions commonly treated by rehabilitation providers.

The World Health Organization (WHO) estimates that approximately 1 billion people, or 15% of the global population, are living with some form of disability.[6] Furthermore, disability prevalence is higher in low- and middle-income countries such as Nepal.[6] As the aging population increases globally, the disability trend is also expected to increase.[7] In addition, a recent prolonged civil war (1996–2006) and frequent natural disasters, including major earthquakes in 2015, have also led to increased impairments and disability in Nepal.

During Nepal's 2011 census, 2% of the country's population reported some kind of disability, defined as the following: "physical disability, blind and low vision, deaf and hard of hearing, deaf-blind, speech problem, mental illness, intellectual disability, and multiple disability."[8] Of these, physical disability accounted for more one-third of the reported disabilities. Following this report, the Central Bureau of Statistics recognized the potential for underreporting of disability during the census and has called for large-scale, dedicated household surveys to be conducted to provide better nationwide statistics on disability. More than half of the individuals with disabilities in Nepal are of economically productive age (15–59 years), and disabilities are similarly prevalent in urban and rural areas.[8]

According to the Institute of Health Metrics and Evaluation, low back pain is the top cause of disability in Nepal, and cardiovascular disease causes the most disability-adjusted life years (DALYs).[1] Nepal's most common causes of disability and DALYs are listed in **Box 1** and **Table 1**, respectively. Although population-based injury data are limited, hospital-based surveillance demonstrates that the most common causes of injuries include falls, road traffic injuries, and burns.[9]

Access to health care in Nepal is limited. According to the Nepal Demographic and Health Survey completed in 2016, 11% of households nationwide have to travel more than 1 hour to reach the nearest government health facility. This percentage disproportionately affects more mountainous regions and poorer households.[10] Looking at rehabilitation services specifically, a recent systematic review of access to rehabilitation for people with disabilities in low- and middle-income countries demonstrated low coverage in general.[11] The authors also identified barriers to rehabilitation including the following: distance to service, availability/cost of transportation, affordability of services, and knowledge and attitude factors specific to the service.[11]

THE CURRENT STATE OF REHABILITATION IN NEPAL
Institutions

At present, there is no government rehabilitation hospital. Although some acute hospitals offer inpatient physiotherapy services, none have dedicated acute rehabilitation units, and none employ physical medicine and rehabilitation consultants.

International nongovernmental organizations (INGOs) and local nongovernmental organizations (NGOs) have played vital roles in developing rehabilitation institutions in Nepal. Three hospitals provide most of the inpatient rehabilitation services for the entire country.

Green Pastures Hospital was originally established in 1957 by the International Nepal Fellowship as a leprosy hospital, and services were subsequently expanded to include

---

Box 1
Health problems causing the most disability in Nepal, in order of rank

1. Cardiovascular disease
2. Maternal and neonatal
3. Chronic respiratory
4. Respiratory infections and tuberculosis
5. Musculoskeletal disorders
6. Neoplasms
7. Mental disorders
8. Neurologic disorders
9. Enteric infections
10. Transport injuries

Data from Viz Hub. Available at: http://vizhub.healthdata.org/gbd-compare.

Table 1		
Top 10 causes of disability-adjusted life years: Nepal 2017		
Rank	Cause	Rate per 100,000
1	Cardiovascular disease	3859
2	Maternal and neonatal	3267
3	Chronic respiratory	2456
4	Respiratory infections and tuberculosis	2238
5	Musculoskeletal disorders	1870
6	Neoplasms	1684
7	Mental disorders	1525
8	Neurologic disorders	1503
9	Enteric infections	1355
10	Transport injuries	1246

Data from Viz Hub. Available at: http://vizhub.healthdata.org/gbd-compare.

individuals with spinal cord injury (SCI), stroke, and traumatic brain injury in the late 1990s. Staff training at the time of expansion was supported and provided by international partners.[12] Currently Green Pastures has 40 inpatient rehabilitation beds, 20 for individuals with leprosy and 20 for individuals with other rehabilitation needs.

The Hospital for Rehabilitation and Disabled Children was conceived by a Nepali orthopedic surgeon, Professor Doctor Ashok K. Banskota, who began offering services to the disabled poor in the 1980s. The center was initially supported by INGOs and is now run by a Nepali NGO. The center has 100 inpatient beds, sees more than 25,000 outpatient visits annually, and runs satellite clinics as part of a comprehensive community-based rehabilitation (CBR) program.

The concept of a Spinal Injury Rehabilitation Center (SIRC) began when a prominent Nepali journalist, Mr Kanak Mani Dixit, sustained a fall-related SCI in 2001 while trekking in the mountains. Mr Dixit, along with a group of colleagues and friends, established a local NGO that founded SIRC in 2002, now Nepal's largest SCI inpatient rehabilitation center. SIRC has 51 inpatient SCI beds and has recently expanded services to include 10 stroke and traumatic brain injury beds. SIRC provides inpatient rehabilitation for approximately 300 individuals with SCI per year and provides outpatient care, home follow-up visits, community outreach programs, and a residential vocational rehabilitation program.

Providers

The rehabilitation workforce is limited in Nepal. There are no training programs for medical doctors to specialize in the internationally recognized field of physical medicine and rehabilitation (PM&R). At present, only one Nepali PM&R doctor is registered with the Nepal Medical Council (NMC) and practicing in the country.

In Nepal, there is 1 physiotherapy school at Kathmandu University of Medical Sciences, which offers a bachelor's degree in physiotherapy. Individuals interested in postgraduate degrees must pursue these studies abroad. Currently, 1524 physiotherapist in different specialization and in different levels are registered with Nepal Health Professional Council (NHPC).

A bachelor's degree in audiology, speech, and language pathology is available through the Institute of Medicine with affiliation to Tribhuvan University; however, only 75 speech and hearing individual providers are registered with NHPC in the entire country.

There are no formal training programs for occupational therapy in Nepal. Although the exact number of occupational therapists in Nepal is unknown, 9 institutions/organizations offer occupational therapy services throughout the country.

Training in prosthetics, orthotics, and/or assistive device technology is also not available in Nepal. 24 individuals with training on the use of prosthetics and orthotics training are registered with NHPC throughout the country.

These obvious workforce limitations have sweeping implications. As the WHO World Report on Disability states, "Unmet rehabilitation needs can delay discharge, limit activities, restrict participation, cause deterioration in health, increase dependency on others for assistance, and decrease quality of life. These negative outcomes can have broad social and financial implications for individuals, families, and communities."[6]

Technology

The availability of assistive devices, including mobility aids, is inadequate; most of them must be imported. Many individuals and institutions rely on outside organizations and donations for these devices. No local manufacturers exist in Nepal to meet the needs of people with impairments and disability.

Policy

The importance of and the need for rehabilitation was brought to the forefront of planning and policy making immediately after the 2015 earthquakes in Nepal. According to the Nepal Government's new Policy, Strategy, and Ten Years Action Plan on Disability Management,[13] finalized in 2016, within 5 years, adequate disability and rehabilitation human resources should be produced and posts created for primary disability identification, management, referral, and counseling. PM&R physicians are included in the required posts. Furthermore, within 10 years every region and state should have at least one fully equipped rehabilitation center and established orthotics/prosthetics workshop. This new policy reflects a commitment from the Nepali government, which ratified the CRPD in 2010, and marks a dramatic improvement in attention and support given to caring for individuals with disabilities and expanding rehabilitation services throughout the country.

FUTURE DIRECTION

Given the significant need for rehabilitation in Nepal and the extremely limited services currently offered, implementation of the Policy, Strategy, and Ten Years Action Plan on Disability Management is imperative. In addition, specific focus should be given to establishing and improving training and education opportunities for rehabilitation providers and broader implementation of multi-/interdisciplinary rehabilitation in health systems nationwide. We focus strongly on developing and improving training opportunities in Nepal, because a recent survey carried out by the International Labor Organization found that nearly 40% of Nepali health care students planned to migrate abroad for further education.[14] Although this study focuses only on medical and nursing students, we have personally witnessed similar trends among physiotherapists at our center.

Rehabilitation Education and Training

We believe that PM&R specialization should be made available to doctors in Nepal as soon as possible. Multiple international partners are ready and willing to provide educational support in the initial stages of PM&R training, and indeed are necessary given the current lack of PM&R physicians. Nepal could and should institute a 3-year PM&R residency with a standardized curriculum that covers the breadth and depth of the field. This curriculum would apply at multiple teaching sites in the country to provide, at a minimum, clinical rotations with academic preceptors in the following areas: SCI rehabilitation, stroke and brain injury rehabilitation, orthopedic rehabilitation, pediatric rehabilitation, wound care, burn rehabilitation, prosthetics and orthotics, electrodiagnosis, and musculoskeletal medicine. Contextual needs, such as leprosy rehabilitation, for example, should be considered in curriculum development.

During the initial years of residency training, local faculty in partnership with visiting international faculty would serve as preceptors to ensure evidence-based education throughout the clinical rotations, as well as standardized assessment and professional licensure/registration. As Nepali PM&R residents graduate and enter independent practice, the regular use of international faculty members can be appropriately phased out and such training will be fully sustained by Nepali PM&R specialists.

In addition, steps should be taken to increase opportunities for physiotherapists to pursue training at postgraduate level in Nepal. We also strongly urge the Ministry of Health and Ministry of Education to take steps to develop graduate and postgraduate occupational therapy as well as prosthetics and orthotics programs.

Health Systems

WHO's recent Rehabilitation in Health Systems recommendations clearly lay out priorities to strengthen rehabilitation in the context of Nepal.[3] **Table 2** presents the strongest evidence-based recommendations made, all of which are at least partially targeted by the government's Action Plan on Disability management.

The implementation of these 3 recommendations alone will significantly improve the quality and coverage of rehabilitation services offered throughout Nepal. Unique to our context is the rugged/mountainous terrain. Given this, and the reality that 80% of the population live in rural communities, providing coordinated CBR services throughout the country is critical.[2] Currently, there are 50 to 60 CBR programs being implemented by local NGOs and organizations. Twelve of these programs are supported by the Ministry of Women, Children and Social Welfare directly, whereas others are supported by NGOs and INGOs. However, no network exists to link these CBR programs. Strong collaboration and coordination among organizations to maximize CBR provision and coverage throughout the country is imperative and needs to be implemented.

Research in Rehabilitation

There is limited research in PM&R in the context of Nepal. Most of the available literature is hospital based and descriptive in nature. Population-based studies are needed to fully understand the prevalence of conditions that lead to the need for

Table 2 WHO recommendations on rehabilitation in health systems	
Recommendation	**Evidence**
A multidisciplinary rehabilitation workforce should be available	High
Both community and hospital rehabilitation services should be available	Moderate
Hospitals should include specialized rehabilitation units for inpatients with complex needs	Very high

Only recommendations with "strong" strength of recommendation are included.
Data from World Health Organization. Rehabilitation in health systems. Available at: http://www.who.int/rehabilitation/rehabilitation_health_systems/en/. Accessed 5 December 2018.

rehabilitation. Consistent with the WHO's recommendations, research priorities in Nepal should focus on cost–benefit analyses of rehabilitation services, rehabilitation access, and measuring the impact of rehabilitation in standardized ways that have been validated in the context of Nepal.[3] In addition, high-quality interventional studies in Nepal and/or similar contexts are needed to improve and maximize rehabilitation efficacy.

SUMMARY

The need for rehabilitation services in Nepal is great. As rehabilitation becomes a more specific focus among stakeholders nationally and globally, now is the time for Nepal to not only plan but also implement evidence-based strategies to provide more comprehensive person-centered rehabilitation that optimizes function and reduces disability. The results will undoubtedly have an impact individuals, families, communities, and indeed the entire country.[3]

REFERENCES

1. Institute for Health Metrics and Evaluation. Nepal Country Profile 2018. Available at: www.healthdata.org/nepal. Accessed December 3, 2018.
2. World Bank. Country Profile: Nepal. 2018. Available at: https://data.worldbank.org/country/nepal. Accessed December 3, 2018.
3. World Health Organization. Rehabilitation in health systems 2017. Available at: http://www.who.int/rehabilitation/rehabilitation_health_systems/en/. Accessed December 5, 2018.
4. United Nations. Convention on the rights of persons with disabilities 2006. Available at: http://www.un.org/disabilities/documents/convention/convoptprot-e.pdf. Accessed December 5, 2018.
5. Kamenov K, Mills JA, Chatterji S, et al. Needs and unmet needs for rehabilitation services: a scoping review. Disabil Rehabil 2019;41(10):1227–37.
6. World Health Organization and World Bank. World report on disability. 2011. Available at: http://www.who.int/disabilities/world_report/2011/en/. Accessed December 5, 2018.
7. United Nations. World population ageing 2015. Available at: http://www.un.org/en/development/desa/population/publications/pdf/ageing/WPA2015_Report.pdf. Accessed December 5, 2018.
8. Government of Nepal Central Bureau of Statistics. National population and housing census 2011. Available at: http://cbs.gov.np/sectoral_statistics/population/national_report. Accessed December 5, 2018.
9. Government of Nepal Ministry of Health. Annual report Department of Health Services 2016/2017. Kathmandu (Nepal): Government of Nepal; 2017. Available at: dohs.gov.np/wp-content/uploads/2018/04/Annual_Report_2073-74.pdf. Accessed December 5, 2018.
10. Ministry of Health NNEal. Nepal Demographic and health survey 2016 2017. Available at: https://www.dhsprogram.com/pubs/pdf/fr336/fr336.pdf. Accessed 3 December 2018.
11. Bright T, Wallace S, Kuper H. A systematic review of access to rehabilitation for people with disabilities in low- and middle-income countries. Int J Environ Res Public Health 2018;15(10) [pii:E2165].
12. Brandsma JW, Schwarz RJ, Anderson AM, et al. Transformation of a leprosy hospital in Nepal into a rehabilitation centre: the Green Pastures Hospital experience. Lepr Rev 2005;76(4):267–76.

13. Government of Nepal Leprosy Control Division. Policy, strategy, and ten years action plan on disability management (2073 - 2083). Kathmandu (Nepal): Government of Nepal Leprosy Control Division; 2016.

14. International Labour Organization. Migration of health workers from Nepal. 2017. Available at: https://ceslam.org/docs/publicationManagement/ILO_Migration_of_Health_Workers_from_Nepal.pdf. Accessed December 5, 2018.

Rehabilitation in Bangladesh

Taslim Uddin, MBBS, FCPS[a],*, Moshiur Rahman Khasru, MBBS, FCPS[a],
Mohammad Tariqul Islam, MBBS, FCPS[a], Mohammad Ali Emran, MBBS, FCPS[a],
Mohammad Shahidur Rahman, MBBS, FCPS[a],
Mohammad Abdus Shakoor, MBBS, FCPS, PhD[a],
Abul Khair Mohammad Salek, MBBS, FCPS[a], Syed Mozaffar Ahmed, MBBS, FCPS[a],
Mohammad Moniruzzaman Khan, MBBS, FCPS[a],
Mohammad Ahsan Ullah, MBBS, FCPS[a], Badrunnesa Ahmed, MBBS, FCPS[a],
Mohammad Nuruzzaman Khandoker, MBBS, FCPS[a],
Farzana Khan Shoma, MBBS, FCPS[a], Mahmudur Rahman, MBBS, FCPS[a],
Shamsun Nahar, MBBS, FCPS[a], Mohammad Habibur Rahman, MBBS, FCPS[b],
Mohammad Moyeenuzzaman, MBBS, FCPS[a]

KEYWORDS

- Disability • Rehabilitation • History • Bangladesh • Training • Medical education

KEY POINTS

- Bangladesh is a developing country with highest population density.
- Current scenario of disability and medical rehabilitation services in Bangladesh is focused in this article.
- Disability rights are emphasized and further improvement of rehabilitation workforce and services are advocated in this manuscript.

INTRODUCTION

There has been notable progress and improvement in the clinical practice and education of physical medicine and rehabilitation (PMR) in Bangladesh since its inception in 1969.[1] Mixed thoughts exist regarding the history and progression of the specialty among physiatrists, other physicians, policy makers, and the patient population. World-wide, the prevalence of disability is increasing in line with the aging population and the global increase in noncommunicable diseases (NCD), mental health, and road traffic

Disclosure Statement: The authors have nothing to disclose.
[a] Department of Physical Medicine and Rehabilitation, Bangabandhu Sheikh Mujib Medical University, Dhaka 1000, Bangladesh; [b] Department of Physical Medicine and Rehabilitation, National Institute of Traumatology and Orthopedic Rehabilitation (NITOR), Sher-E-Bangla Nagar, Dhaka 1207, Bangladesh
* Corresponding author.
E-mail address: taslimpmr@gmail.com

injuries. Bangladesh, as 1 of the 194 United Nations member states, endorsed the World Health Organization (WHO) global disability action plan (GDAP) 2014 to 2021.[2,3] The highlights of the objectives of the GDAP are to remove barriers and improve access to health services, strengthen health-related rehabilitation with community-based rehabilitation, and enhance the collection of disability-related information and research on disability and related services. There is an increasing unmet need for rehabilitation, particularly in less economically developed countries, highlights in the call for action by WHO Rehabilitation 2030.[4] More attention is required to achieve safe rehabilitation practice with protection for the patients and rehabilitation team members. At the same time, future physiatrists and other rehabilitation associates need to be guided in line with national and international demands. This article reports on existing knowledge on the entity and principles of assessment of rehabilitation services, and identification and analysis of the potential opportunities and challenges of medical rehabilitation in Bangladesh, with comments on avenues of improvement.

METHODS

The information used in this article was collected from multiple sources. This included an online English literature search, with predetermined key words, of official web pages related to disability and medical rehabilitation, and interviews with senior PMR physicians, related government officials, and other rehabilitation professionals. Published hard copies of PMR conference proceedings were also consulted. Data and figures were further checked during supplementary group discussions at the Bangladesh PMR executive body meeting, 2018. A special workshop session was organized during the Bangladesh Association of Physical Medicine and Rehabilitation conference (BAPMRCON) 2018, facilitated by the lead author of this article, to highlight opportunities and challenges in the development of PMR in Bangladesh, which was attended by PMR faculties from Bangladesh, the Royal Melbourne Hospital of Australia, and DC University Hospital of South Korea.

Complementary input was also welcomed from the Institutional Quality Assurance Cell and Self-Assessment Committee (SAC) of PMR, Bangabandhu Sheikh Mujib Medical University (BSMMU), after conducting a survey with structured questionnaires among different stakeholders of PMR from January 2018 to May 2018. The SAC committee finalized their improvement plan after review by an external peer review team, with the aim of improving patient care services and PMR medical education.

The online literature search involved articles from 1960 to 2018 with predefined key words in BanglaJol, Google Scholar, and Medline restricted to the English language. Keywords used were (but not limited to) Bangladesh, developing countries, disability, medical rehabilitation, neurorehabilitation, disaster medical rehabilitation, physiotherapy, occupational therapy, speech and language therapy, and prosthetics and orthotics (P&O). Boolean logic was used to generate different combinations of search strings.

Identified opportunities and challenges in the development of rehabilitation services are listed in **Box 1**.

BANGLADESH HEALTH INDEX

Bangladesh is a developing country covering an area of 147,000 km^2 and has a population of 1.67 million. This is equivalent to 2.18% of the total world population, ranking eighth in the list of countries by population with 1278 persons/km^2; 36.5% of the population live in urban areas, and the median age is 26.0 years.[5]

Box 1
Opportunities and challenges

- Opportunities
  - PMR physicians are popular among patients
  - Huge number of varied patients: 500 per day in BSMMU OPDs
  - Physiatrist is a leader and keen to work
  - Popular specialty among new medical graduates
  - Early expert career exposure to procedures and interventions with friendly faculties
  - Early exposure to procedures and independent consultation by the trainees in PMR
  - Internationally recognized Bangladesh PMR
  - Connectivity with expatriate physiatrists
  - Collaboration for training and research with other institutes and NGOs
  - Public and private partnership in rehabilitation, for example, developing autistic schools, disability welfare society

- Weaknesses and challenges
  - Lack of information about disability and medical rehabilitation in Bangladesh
  - Inadequate system of identification and surveillance of disability
  - Fewer PMR specialists and skilled rehabilitation professionals
  - Fewer female physiatrists and other rehabilitation professionals
  - Fewer posts at government, private, and nongovernment levels
  - Minimal or no undergraduate PMR exposure
  - Limited number of quality PMR training centers for SCI, TBI, P&O, amputee, and rehabilitation service outlets
  - Limited research activities by senior physiatrists covering different areas of rehabilitation
  - Serious space crisis for expansion
  - Lack of good governance and interference by others
  - Poor system of punishment and provision of rewards
  - Placement of funds
  - Poor interdepartmental relationships
  - Persons other than medical experts are the final decision makers in health services

---

The male-to-female ratio is approximately 1:1. More than 53.7% of the population are of reproductive age (15 to 49 years), 30.8% are children (0 to 14 years), and 16.3% are 50 years or older. The population growth rate is 1.37%, the birth rate is 18.8 births per 1000 population, and the mortality rate is 5.1 deaths per 1000 population.[6]

The literacy rate is 63.6% and is increasing gradually. Currently, Bangladesh holds first place in South Asia, second place in Asia, and 47th position across the globe in the Global Gender Equality Index. Approximately 95% of the population speak Bengali; the majority are Muslims (86.6%), followed by Hindus (12.1%), Buddhists (0.6%), Christians (0.4%), and other religions (0.3%). The current gross domestic product (GDP) is $1602, the GDP growth rate is 7.64%, and the poverty level is 23.5%. Bangladesh ranks 139th in the Human Development Index.[7]

The health care system run by the public and private sectors by local entrepreneurs, different nongovernment organizations (NGOs), and international organizations. In the public sector, the Ministry of Health and Family Welfare is the leading organization for policy formulation, planning, and decision making at macro and micro levels. Under the ministry, 4 directorates, namely Directorate General of Health Services, Directorate General of Family Planning, Directorate of Nursing Services, and Directorate General of Drug Administration, provide health care services to the citizens.

CURRENT SITUATION OF DISABILITY AND THE DISABLED IN BANGLADESH

The WHO World Report on Disability estimates that 15% of the world's population has some form of disability, citing Bangladesh as a low-income developing country with more than 20 million people living with disability[8]; more specifically, 10% of the population have significant disabilities in mobility and performing self-care daily living activities at home and in workplaces.[9] Few reliable data are available on disability prevalence and its impact in Bangladesh. The Bangladesh Bureau of Statistics (BBS), as the pertinent government organization, oversaw national censuses[10] in 1981, 1991, and 2001, and some other private organizations conducted surveys to determine disability prevalence, as shown in **Table 1**. The statistics on the prevalence of disability has been a matter of serious debate. Most of the estimates of disability prevalence generally seem to be underrated, sometimes excessively. Thus, disability prevalence is estimated as 9.0%, but ranges from 0.47% to 14.4% in different studies.[10]

Disability in specific age and gender categories, such as children and women, are important as a reflection of inequality. UNICEF reported a disability prevalence range from 1.4% to 17.5% in 2014. A higher ratio of disability is reported in females, the older population, and rural residents.[11–13]

Types of Disability

The spectrum of disabilities[14] is classified in the Bangladesh Disability Rights and Protection Act 2013, as listed in **Table 2**. Physical, psychosocial, visual, speech, intellectual, hearing, and hearing-visual disability, autism, cerebral palsy, Down syndrome, and multiple disabilities all exist in Bangladesh, of which physical disability[15] is the most prevalent (22.5%).

Disability Impact

In 2014, a study by Ali[16] found that the cumulative cost of 4 components, namely, (1) costs arising from lack of access to employment, (2) costs attributable to children with disabilities losing out on school, (3) costs incurred by adults helping people with disabilities, and (4) costs for children helping a family member with disabilities, is approximately US $1.18 billion per year, which equates to about 1.74% of Bangladesh's GDP. Religious issues also influence disability by preventing inclusiveness.[17]

Table 1
Disability prevalence based on census and/or survey

	Organization with Year of Survey/Report	Prevalence (%)
Census/survey based on Government of Bangladesh organization	BBS census 1981	0.82
	BBS census 1991	0.47
	BBS census 2001	0.60
	BBS disability prevalence survey 1994	1.06
	BBS survey 2009	1.00
	BBS survey 2010	1.18
	BBS HIES 2010	9.07
Census/survey based on private organization	Action Aid baseline survey 1995–1997 (in 4 locations)	14.4
	Action Aid baseline survey 1995–1997 (in 5 locations)	13.34
	The Innovators KAP Survey 2005	6.0
	ESCAP 2012	9.0
UUNICEF	UNICEF cited 2014	1.4–17.5

Table 2 Types of disability	
Type of Disability	**Percentage**
Physical	22.5
Visual	13.7
Hearing	16.8
Intellectual	10.1
Mental	12.8
Others	24.2

Rehabilitation Team Functioning

Intensive rehabilitation requires a dedicated team of skilled professionals facilitated and guided by a physiatrist. However, teamwork previously was lacking in Bangladeshi rehabilitation practice. Recently, a functioning team started activities at BSMMU, comprising a physiotherapist (PT), occupational therapist (OT), speech language therapist (SLT), rehabilitating nurse, nutritionist, P&O specialist, and residents from psychiatry facilitated by senior faculties of rehabilitation and PMR residents. There is a lack of proper knowledge about medical rehabilitation and its jurisdiction among physicians of other disciplines, and ideas that used to be conceived (practiced) by physicians decades ago are still in practice among some of today's doctors, who understand physiotherapy merely as a "total rehab" endeavor. Even musculoskeletal physicians (orthopedists, rheumatologists, and neurologists) are not properly maintaining interdisciplinary relationships with rehabilitation team members.

PHYSIATRY IN BANGLADESH

The first-generation pioneer physiatrists, namely Professors Wahid, Hossian, and Quamrul Islam, were trained and graduated at the Royal College of Physicians (United Kingdom) during the 1960s. Of these 3 physiatrists, Quamrul Islam joined as assistant professor in Dhaka Medical College during 1969 and started the new specialty of physical medicine (PM). Through the dynamic leadership of Professor Islam, PM has gained momentum with the introduction of Fellowship (FCPS) and Doctor of Medicine (MD) courses in 1989 and 1998, respectively. Residency training courses (MD) started during 2005 at BSMMU and at Dhaka Medical College in 2010. These courses are run by 2 different authorities, and BSMMU is working as the center of excellence for PMR teaching and training in Bangladesh. Enrollment in the courses is through a nationwide and highly competitive examination.

Effective from 2001, PM has been updated to PMR, with an office order of the Ministry of Health and Family Welfare. As of July 2018, 133 physiatrists have completed their postgraduation in PMR and are serving for the betterment of people with disability and their rehabilitation at home and abroad, with good reputations.

In Bangladesh, rehabilitation practices vary in different settings, and the possibility of total rehabilitation under one roof is lacking. Several institutions, namely BSMMU, Chittagong Medical College Hospital, Dhaka Medical College Hospital, Shaheed Suhrawardi Medical College Hospital, and the Armed Forces Rehabilitation Center at Dhaka, are currently operating reputably. PMR physicians need to maintain a standard uniform continuum of care for persons with disability (PwD) to prevent confusion among other physicians and patients' families. Most PMR practices are related to pain or the musculoskeletal (MSK) system. The rehabilitation field is also required to cover disabilities resulting from brain injury, spinal cord injury, as well as amputee rehabilitation and much more.

Currently, 2 institutions provide postgraduation education in PMR, namely the Bangladesh College of Physicians and Surgeons (BCPS) and the BSMMU. Other therapy professionals graduate from public and private universities with BSc degrees and diplomas.

1. BCPS was formed[18] in 1972 as the highest body for conferring postgraduate qualifications in various disciplines of medical science. The postgraduation degree offered by BCPS is FCPS (Fellow of the College of Physicians and Surgeons). FCPS has 2 parts, I and II. Candidates are eligible for entry to the FCPS Part I examination 18 months after completion of their medical degree (MBBS). Requisites for undertaking the part II examination are (a) successfully passing the part I examination, (b) completion of 3 years of semistructured training in an accredited center or 2 years of training in an accredited center plus 1 year of course work in the subjects, and (c) production of a research report of acceptable quality in the form of a dissertation.

2. BSMMU[19–21]BSMMU is the first public medical university in Bangladesh, established in 1998. The university offers courses such as MD, PhD, MS, MPhil, MDS, and a diploma. It bears the heritage of the Institute of Postgraduate Medical Research, established in December 1965. It has an enviable reputation for providing high-quality postgraduate education in different specialties. However, courses for rehabilitation team professionals such as PT, OT, SLT, P&O, and others are lacking.

Residency, as a competency-based program, is for 5 years and includes 2 phases, described in **Box 2**.

Box 2
Course curriculum for MD phase A and B in physical medicine and rehabilitation

Phase A

Two years' duration divided into 8 blocks, aims at a broad-based training in general physical medicine and rehabilitation as the foundation of PMR and allied specialties, including internal medicine, rheumatology, neurology, orthopedic surgery, pediatrics, geriatrics, cardiology, critical care medicine, and respiratory medicine. After completion, the residents undertake a summative examination before being promoted to phase B.

Phase B

PMR comprehensive and structured 3-year course. Special emphasis on rehabilitation of patients with stroke, geriatrics, MSK, traumatic brain injury, spinal cord injury, and cardiopulmonary disorders. Electrodiagnostic medicine, for example, EMG-NCV, I-T curve, and MSK ultrasonography, is also highlighted.

Residents perform academic activities alongside primary responsibilities to treat the patients under direct supervision of the faculty.

As part of this course, the residents need to prepare a thesis under the guidance of a recognized supervisor. They are required to present the thesis and undertake summative written, objective structured practical, clinical, and oral examinations before they are awarded the MD degree.

REHABILITATION TRAINING

Table 3 describes postgraduate courses mainly confined to BSMMU and DMCH, although training is recognized in other institutions as already mentioned. Faculties and allied professional facilities are limited in comparison with other countries.[15,22]

Course content is not updated regularly, and the curriculum is not designed as such. Hence, at the end of the session, some of topics are not discussed. The examination schedule is strict regarding the January and June sessions.

Training rotations for inpatients as discussed in **Box 2** require the Incorporation of International Classification of Functioning disabilities and Health (ICF) as the core set of rehabilitation in the training programs, as prioritized by Stucki[23] and the European Union of Medical Specialists in 2005.

Programs lack adequate exposure to human motion analysis gait laboratories, electrodiagnostic medicine, sports medicine, geriatric medicine, and pediatric rehabilitation, as well as special inpatient rehabilitation programs for brain injury, cardiac rehabilitation, vestibular system and balance, amputation, and spinal cord injury. There is a serious crisis of space in almost all of the departments where the trainees rotate.

Training for the residents and fellowship courses are also deficient in structured programs on orthotics, prosthetics, assistive devices, and robotics. However, they have an impressive exposure to musculoskeletal medicine, rheumatology-related pain management, including interventional pain management, and outpatient management of chronic disabilities. The trainees learn skills under the direct supervision of a unit head with different practice styles and settings in rotation blocks, ultimately enriching their insight on physiatrist practice as a future PMR leader.

This program is consistent with the revised definition of physiatry[24] dealing with PMR, musculoskeletal pain medicine, and neurorehabilitation.

The residents work hard, learn a lot, and enjoy the work. They participate in disability-related and rehabilitation-related special calendar days, and social and continued medical education programs.

Individual components of the evaluation system (written, clinical, and oral), which run the possibility of repetitions and omissions, require extensive revision. At the

Table 3
Current strength of physical medicine and rehabilitation academic staff and allies

Institution	Faculty	Medical Officer	Residents and Trainee	PT	OT	SLT
BSMMU	14	12	39	13	1	1
DMCH	5	6	21	10	1	1
CMCH	5	6	6	10	–	–
ShSMCH	5	6	6	8	–	–
SSMCH	2	4	2	8	–	–
NINS	3	4	2	8	–	1
NITOR	3	4	4	10	2	–
BIRDEM	2	4	2	6	–	–

Abbreviations: BIRDEM, Bangladesh Institute of Research and Rehabilitation in Diabetes, Endocrine and Metabolic Disorders; BSMMU, Bangabandhu Sheikh Mujib Medical University; CMCH, Chittagong Medical College Hospital; DMCH, Dhaka Medical College Hospital; NINS, National Institute of Neurosciences & Hospital; NITOR, National Institute of Traumatology and Orthopedic Rehabilitation; OT, occupational therapist; PT, physiotherapist; ShSMCH, Shaheed Suhrawardy Medical College Hospital; SLT, speech and language therapist; SSMCH, Sir Salimullah Medical College Hospital.

end of the training programs, the residents successfully acquire the specified physiatrist degree, with minimal dropout rate. At the same time, they need to acquire the 5 most important quality aspects of physiatrist training: being a good listener, translator, manager, and innovative and tolerant for uncertainty, as suggested by Weinstein.[25]

OTHER REHABILITATION PROFESSIONALS IN BANGLADESH

PMR is multidisciplinary and entails the services of other rehabilitation professionals. A summary of the current status of rehabilitation professions is shown in **Table 4**. The Bangladesh Physiotherapy Association (BPA) is the main representative body for Bangladeshi physical therapists (PTs).[26] There are an estimated 2400 PTs in the country. The training programs in PT include a 3-year diploma, a 4-year bachelor degree, and a masters program. According to the Bangladesh Occupational Therapy Association (BOTA),[27] 250 OTs have graduated from the Center for the Rehabilitation of the Paralyzed (CRP). An estimated 260 graduate SLTs are currently in Bangladesh (Ms Sanjida Akter, Secretary of Speech and Language therapists Association in Bangladesh, personal communication, October 2018). The opportunities for therapy professionals are limited. Most of them are working in the private health care sector, some are employed under the Ministry of Social welfare, a few are working in government sectors, and others are working with NGOs.

RESEARCH AND ETHICAL ISSUES

The trends in research by PMR physicians in Bangladesh are mostly pain related. Of 197 PMR dissertations and theses identified, 72% of research topics involved therapy modality or were related to musculoskeletal system diseases (BCPS web page at https://bcps.edu.bd/, BSMMU Library). OPD-based retrospective studies are performed in a national neurology hospital where patients primarily attend for neurologic consultations. The disease patterns and demographic information of the patients are an indication of the kind of patients who are attending. Research in rehabilitation after disasters and in austere environments are also important aspects presented by physiatrists in Bangladesh.[28]

There are few epidemiologic research studies on spinal cord injury rehabilitation by the CRP.[29] Quality research is required in robotic rehabilitation, assistive technology, rehabilitation engineering, and stem cell technology. Physiatrists, as leaders of health-related rehabilitation in a multidisciplinary field, are trained in interventional physiatry

Table 4
Overview of other rehabilitation professionals in Bangladesh

Professional Category	Representative Organization in Bangladesh	Estimated Number in Bangladesh	Degree Courses Available
PT	BPA	2400	Graduate (4 y) and diploma (3 y)
OT	BOTA	250	Graduate (4 y) under Dhaka University
SLT	Speech and Language Therapists Association	260	Graduate (4 y) under Dhaka University

Abbreviations: BOTA, Bangladesh Occupational Therapy Association; BPA, Bangladesh Physiotherapy Association; OT, occupational therapist; PT, physiotherapist; SLT, speech and language therapist.

to perform intramuscular and intra-articular injections as well as nerve conduction studies.[30] Research in various interventions, especially ultrasound-guided and fluoroscopy-guided interventions, are also necessary because many physiatrists are required to carry out such procedures. Recently, a relatively younger group started regenerative medicine research in medical rehabilitation.[31] Evidence indicates that goal setting may lead to a higher quality of life for the person with disability, in this context reducing the possibility of rehospitalization or death.[32] There is an urgent need for research directed toward rehabilitation goal setting, low-cost techniques of disability evaluation, and clinical, home-based, and community-based rehabilitation.

SUMMARY

Disability remains a neglected issue and PwD face multiple barriers, although progress in health care systems in Bangladesh is taking place. There is a need to collect large-scale epidemiologic data on disability and to enforce disability legislation countrywide. PMR physicians need to take a leadership role in a functioning rehabilitation team. Physiatrists, in collaboration with other rehabilitation professionals, can help provide comprehensive rehabilitation services for PwD in Bangladesh. Rehabilitation services should be strengthened to include improved training and job opportunities for PMR physicians and other rehabilitation professionals. To sustain the growing trend in health indices, medical rehabilitation services at the community level need to be urgently implemented to ensure a better future and quality of life for PwD in Bangladesh.

ACKNOWLEDGMENTS

No financial involvement and conflicts of interest was implicated. However, the authors would like to acknowledge consultants, PMR residents and fellows of BSMMU as well as to Dr Hasan Tasdeed Mohammad for data management.

REFERENCES

1. Bangladesh Association of Physical Medicine and Rehabilitation (BAPMR). Available at: http://www.bapmr.org.bd. Accessed October 16, 2018.
2. UN Statistics on Bangladesh. Available at: http://www.un.int/bangladesh. Accessed November 28, 2018.
3. World Health Organization. WHO global disability action plan 2014-2015. Better health for all people with a disability. Geneva (Switzerland): WHO Press; 2015. Available at: https://www.who.int/disabilities/actionplan/en/. Accessed October 20, 2018.
4. WHO rehabilitation 2030: a call for action, executive boardroom, WHO headquarters. Geneva (Switzerland), Available at: http://www.who.int/disabilities/care/rehab-2030/en/. Accessed October 20, 2019.
5. Available at: http://www.worldometers.info/world-population/bangladesh-population/. Accessed November 26, 2018.
6. Bangladesh Bureau of Statistics. Available at: http://www.bbs.gov.bd. Accessed November 22, 2018.
7. Bangladesh Economic Review- 2017. Available at: https://mof.gov.bd. Accessed November 22, 2018.
8. World Health Organization. World report on disability. Geneva (Switzerland): WHO; 2006.
9. World Health Organization. Promoting access to health care services for persons with disabilities. Geneva (Switzerland): WHO; 2006.

10. Bangladesh Bureau of Statistics (BBS), Statistics and Informatics Division (SID), Ministry of Planning, Government of People's Republic of Bangladesh. Disability of Bangladesh: prevalence and pattern. Population Monograph 2015;5:30–4.

11. UNICEF Bangladesh. Situation analysis on children with disabilities in Bangladesh. 2014. Available at: https://www.unicef.org/bangladesh/SACDB_Report_FINAL.pdf. Accessed June 07, 2018.

12. Tareque MI, Begum S, Saito Y. Inequality in disability in Bangladesh. PLoS One 2014;9(7):e103681.

13. Quinn ME, Hunter CL, Ray S, et al. The double burden: barriers and facilitators to socioeconomic inclusion for women with disability in Bangladesh. Disability, CBR & Inclusive Development 2016;27(2):128–49. Available at: http://dcidj.org/article/view/474. Accessed November 30, 2018.

14. World Health Organization. Country health profile: Bangladesh. Geneva (Switzerland): WHO; 2015.

15. Khan F, Amatya B, Sayed TM, et al. World Health Organisation global disability action plan 2014-2021: challenges and perspectives for physical medicine and rehabilitation in Pakistan. J Rehabil Med 2017;49:10–21.

16. Ali Z. Economic costs of disability in Bangladesh. Bangladesh Development Studies 2014;XXXVII(4):17–32.

17. Rathore FA, New PW, Iftikhar A. A report on disability and rehabilitation medicine in Pakistan: past, present, and future directions. Arch Phys Med Rehabil 2011; 92(1):161–6.

18. Bangladesh College of Physicians and Surgeons. Syllabus for FCPS-I & FCPS-II physical medicine and rehabilitation. Dhaka: Bangladesh College of Physicians and Surgeons; 2004.

19. Bangabandhu Sheikh Mujib Medical University (BSMMU). Available at: www.bsmmu.edu.bd. Accessed November 27, 2018.

20. Residency Program, Doctor of Medicine (MD). Curriculum (phase A) physical medicine and rehabilitation. Dhaka (Bangladesh): Faculty of Medicine, Bangabandhu Sheikh Mujib Medical University; 2013.

21. Residency Program, Doctor of Medicine (MD). Curriculum (phase B) physical medicine and rehabilitation. Dhaka (Bangladesh): Faculty of Medicine, Bangabandhu Sheikh Mujib Medical University; 2013.

22. Khan F, Amatya B, de Groote W, et al. Capacity-building in clinical skills of rehabilitation workforce in low- and middle-income countries. J Rehabil Med 2018;50: 472–9.

23. Stucki G. International classification of functioning, disability, and health (ICF): a promising framework and classification for rehabilitation medicine. Am J Phys Med Rehabil 2005;84:733–40. Available at: https://doi.org/10.1097/01.phm.0000179521.70639.83. Accessed October 29, 2018.

24. Lee PKW. Defining physiatry and future scopes of rehabilitation medicine. Ann Rehabil Med 2011;35:445–9.

25. Weinstein SM. Defining physiatry: a tolerance for uncertainty. PM R 2011;3:1–2.

26. Bangladesh Physiotherapy Association. Available at: https://www.bpa-bd.org/index.php/2016-12-01-05-08-08/2016-12-01-06-29-31/head-office. Accessed November 19, 2018.

27. Bangladesh Occupational Therapy Association. Available at: http://www.bota.org.bd/contact.php. Accessed November 10, 2018.

28. Uddin T, Islam T, Goseny J Jr. 2017 Bangladesh landslides: physical rehabilitation perspective. Ann Phys Rehabil Med 2018;61(Supplement):e520. Available at: https://doi.org/10.1016/j.rehab.2018.05.1210. Accessed November 30, 2018.

29. Rahman A, Ahmed S, Sultana R, et al. Epidemiology of spinal cord injury in Bangladesh: a five year observation from a rehabilitation center. J Spine 2017; 6:367.
30. Lee PKW. Defining physiatry and future scope of rehabilitation medicine. Ann Rehabil Med 2011;35:445–9.
31. Khasru MR, Salek AKM, Marzen T, et al. Pain and functional outcome with cartilage regeneration in patients with knee osteoarthritis after autologous adipose tissue-derived stem cells therapy: a phase II RCT. Osteoporos Int 2018; 29(Suppl 1):377.
32. Levack WMM, Weatherall M, Hay-Smith EJC, et al. Goal setting and strategies to enhance goal pursuit for adults with acquired disability participating in rehabilitation. Cochrane Database Syst Rev 2015;(7):CD009727. https://doi.org/10.1002/14651858.CD009727.pub2.

Rehabilitation in Malaysia

Amaramalar Selvi Naicker, MBBS, MRehab Med, CIME[a],*,
Saari Mohamad Yatim, MD, MRehab Med[b],
Julia Patrick Engkasan, MBBS, MRehab Med, PhD[c],
Mazlina Mazlan, MBBS, MRehab Med, CMIA[c], Yusniza Mohd. Yusof, MBBS, MRehab Med[d],
Brenda Saria Yuliawiratman, MBBS, MRehab Med, CMIA[a],
Nazirah Hasnan, MBBS, MRehab Med, PhD[c], Ohnmar Htwe, MBBS, MMedSc (Rehab Med), CMIA[a]

KEYWORDS

- People with disabilities • Rehabilitation • Policies • Implementation strategies
- Malaysia

KEY POINTS

- This article reviews the epidemiology, rehabilitation intervention strategies, and rehabilitation resources for persons with disabilities (PWD) in Malaysia.
- Currently, the registered number of PWD is 409,269 individuals, which is 1.3% of the total population, which is far less than the World Health Organization estimation of 10%.
- The rehabilitation implementation strategies include health policies, health promotion, and prevention programs.
- Health-related services for PWD are provided by many government agencies, including health, welfare, education, manpower, housing as well as the private sector and nongovernment organizations.
- It is hoped the national health programs can ensure special care and rehabilitation for PWD while optimizing their self-reliance and social integration.

INTRODUCTION

Rehabilitation in Malaysia was pioneered by expatriates who brought physiotherapy to Malaysia in the 1960s. The first physiotherapy department was established in Kuala Lumpur General Hospital. Although disability care in Malaysia has substantially improved over the past 20 years, people with disability are still subjected to manifold

Disclosure Statement: The authors have nothing to disclose.
[a] Rehabilitation Medicine Unit, Department of Orthopedic and Traumatology, Faculty of Medicine, University Kebangsaan Malaysia, Jalan Yaacob Latif, Bandar Tun Razak, Cheras, Kuala Lumpur 56000, Malaysia; [b] Department of Rehabilitation Medicine, Hospital Serdang, Jalan Puchong, Kajang 43000, Selangor Darul Ehsan, Malaysia; [c] Department of Rehabilitation Medicine, Faculty of Medicine, University of Malaya, Kuala Lumpur 50603, Malaysia; [d] Department of Rehabilitation Medicine, Hospital Rehabilitasi Cheras, Jalan Yaakob Latif, Bandar Tun Razak, Cheras, Kuala Lumpur 56000, Malaysia
* Corresponding author.
E-mail address: asnaicker@yahoo.com

Phys Med Rehabil Clin N Am 30 (2019) 807–816
https://doi.org/10.1016/j.pmr.2019.07.006
1047-9651/19/© 2019 Elsevier Inc. All rights reserved.
pmr.theclinics.com

barriers in their daily encounters. After years of lobbying by various disability organizations, the Persons with Disabilities Act came into effect in 2008 in Malaysia. The Act provides "for the registration, protection, rehabilitation, development and well-being of persons with disabilities and the establishment of the National Council for Persons with Disabilities."[1] The Malaysian Disability Act 2008 defines persons with disabilities (PWD) as those who have long-term physical, mental, intellectual, or sensory impairments, which in interaction with various barriers may hinder their full and effective participation in society. Seven categories of disabilities were recorded, which are vision, hearing, speech, physical, mental, learning difficulties, and multiple disabilities.

At an international level, Malaysia's commitment to care for its disabled members is further reiterated by being a signatory to the Biwako Millennium Framework for Action under the Asia Pacific Decade of the Disabled 2003 to 2012 and the Convention on the Right of Persons with Disabilities 2006 to 2016.[2]

EPIDEMIOLOGY OF DISABILITY IN MALAYSIA

Information on disability prevalence in Malaysia was collected through various sources. One of the main sources of information is from the Population and Housing Census through the "Households Information" category, which is carried out every 10 years. The last one was in 2010 by the Department of Statistics of Malaysia (DOSM).[3] Apart from DOSM, other sources of disability data were from the Department of Social Welfare (DSW), Ministry of Education, Ministry of Health (MOH), nongovernment organizations (NGOs), and other agencies. DSW is responsible for the official registration of people with disabilities and issued detailed guidelines for assessment and certification of various disabilities in 2009. They had also developed a dedicated Disability Information Management System Sistem Pengurusan Maklumat Orang Kurang Upaya (SMOKU) in August 2011 to hasten disability registration and Disability Card distribution.[4]

From the DSW Web site, a total of 409,269 individuals registered as disabled in Malaysia in 2016. This amount is about 1.3% of total Malaysian population of 31.7 million. Learning and physical disabilities accounted for 35% of total disabilities. Visual, mental, and hearing disabilities accounted for 9.0%, 8.2%, and 7.8%, respectively, followed by multiple disabilities (4.7%) and speech (0.5%). Visual and physical disabilities were higher among people aged 60 years and older. Learning disabilities was the highest category reported in children aged 18 years and younger when compared with other categories at 71.7%.[5] As Malaysia is a multiethnic nation, disabilities were seen across all 3 major ethnicities in proportion to its population ratios.

Another major source of disability data was from the MOH, who conduct the National Health and Morbidity Survey regularly. The latest survey in 2015 looked at disability among adults and targeted Malaysian residents in noninstitutionalized living quarters in both urban and rural areas. The prevalence of disability in this study[6] was 3.3% with an estimated 672,529 of the population affected. This amount is higher that the findings of the DSW statistics that had registered a little more than 400,000 members. The prevalence of disability increased with age, with the highest among those aged 61 years or older. The prevalence was also noted to be higher in women than men and in rural compared with urban areas.

The World Health Organization (WHO) estimates 10% to 15% of a country's population would have a disability, which would translate to a minimum of 3.0 million disabled people in a population of 31.7 million in Malaysia. However, the registered number of PWD with the DSW as well as numbers reflected by the National Health and Morbidity Survey 2015 is far below expectations.

Challenges in obtaining the true statistical data on disability in Malaysia are varied.

The negative attitude of PWD toward disability is one of the main factors. Also, disability registration is a voluntary process in Malaysia, and the hesitancy to register is possibly due to fear of stigmatization. Reluctance in respondents to answer surveys on functional limitation and disability was noted, and also the lack of experience of the enumerators has resulted in lower prevalence than estimated by the WHO. Furthermore, lack of knowledge of the public and health professionals on disability and functional impairment is due to limited training and exposure on the topic of disability in medical curriculum in the past. Often doctors are left with their own interpretation of disability and what the person needs. Another major challenge is poor accessibility to register with DSW, and even the online system developed (SMOKU) still requires PWD to be physically present in order to complete the registration and obtain the Disability Card.[7]

REHABILITATION IMPLEMENTATION STRATEGIES

The stakeholders in the provision of services for PWDs include the ministries providing for health, welfare, education, work, transport, housing, arts, and sports. The demands for these services have increased with an increase in awareness about PWDs and the move from charity-based services to the rights-based services.

The need for rehabilitation services has increased rapidly with the improvements in perinatal care (which has resulted in increased survival rates for children with disabilities), change in the demographic structure of the population (a higher proportion of the elderly with increased life expectancy), changes in lifestyle (resulting in increased numbers of persons with chronic diseases and disabilities) as well as violence, depression, and road traffic accidents.

HEALTH POLICIES, HEALTH PROMOTION, AND PREVENTION PROGRAMS

In 1996, the MOH developed the National Health Program and Plan of Action (POA) for the Health Care of PWDs. As a follow-up, several implementation policies and plans were developed, including Health Care for Children with Special Need (1998), Prevention and Control of Blindness (2000) and Deafness (2003), Sexual and Reproductive Health for Children and Adolescent with Disabilities (2004), and Strengthening of Rehabilitation Services at the Health Clinic (2004).

Before that, services in the primary health care were focused more on disability prevention through various immunization programs.

Since 1996, MOH has developed health education materials focusing on specific disabilities, such as cerebral palsy, Down syndrome, and the prevention of deafness and blindness, and has been working with the DSW and NGOs in promotion campaigns, such as the Deaf Awareness Week, Sight for Kid, and celebration of PWD Day.

An early intervention program for children was initiated in 1986 in health clinics. Any child aged 0 to 6 years with any abnormality will be referred to a specialist in hospital. The child health record from 0 to 6 years with guided developmental assessment checklist and health education for parents were meant to empower parents and caregivers to recognize a delay in development and to seek help.

Early detection and prompt treatment can reduce the morbidities leading to disabilities. Programs that work toward prevention of disabilities include antenatal/postnatal care, child health assessment, school health, immunization, nutrition, injury prevention, and healthy lifestyle.

Health and health-related services for PWD are provided by many government agencies, including health, welfare, education, manpower, housing, and so on, and nongovernmental, that is, the private sector and NGOs.

A Malaysian health care program especially for PWD is currently in its second phase (2011–2020) with its POA on Health Care for PWDs. It ensures a comprehensive health care for PWDs. The specific objectives of the POA are to provide equal opportunities for health care, to empower individuals, families, and communities for self-care, and for the development of support services and adequate medical rehabilitation services at all levels of care.

The strategies identified to meet the specific objectives of the plan of action include the following:

1. Advocate on issues and policies of PWDs
2. Increase accessibility to facilities and services
3. Empower individuals, families, and communities
4. Strengthen intersectoral collaboration
5. Ensure adequate and competent workforce
6. Intensify research and development
7. Health program development for specific disabilities

This national health program is planned to meet the current and future needs of PWD, to ensure the right to special care and rehabilitation, to help them enjoy a full and decent life with dignity, and to achieve the greatest degree of self-reliance and social integration.[8,9]

HUMAN RESOURCE AND GOVERNMENT HEALTH CARE FACILITIES

Rehabilitation services delivered by physiotherapists (PT) and occupational therapists (OT) have been operating in government hospitals for decades before 2000. Services focused mainly on physical rehabilitation of mobility and activities of daily living. Of the 1467 PTs, 297 (20%) are placed in 217 health care clinics throughout the country, whereas the remainder are placed in 132 hospitals under the MOH, with another 25 seconded to various governmental agencies, namely the DSW and the Department of Defense.

On the other hand, there are 1217 OTs services, of which 217 (18%) are being placed in the various government outpatient clinics, and the rest are based in hospitals under MOH, while another 29 are seconded to various governmental agencies.

In 1996, the government through MOH first developed a plan of action aimed to develop health services in primary health care for PWD. With this, rehabilitation of the disabled patients is provided not only in hospitals but also in primary care facilities. Currently, there are 242 health centers providing rehabilitation services for children with special needs, 27 health clinics for psychosocial rehabilitative services for stable patients, and 685 health clinics providing rehabilitation for elderly. Placement of PT and OT has witnessed an increase since 2003, and currently, there are 515 therapists in primary health clinics.

Rehabilitative services have been provided in almost all MOH hospitals by PTs and OTs as well as nurses, who form the backbone of rehabilitative service mainly for children in health clinics. The relatively new specialist services in rehabilitation medicine add another dimension and depth toward the care of PWD with the aim of optimizing the functional capacity of an individual despite their disability and reducing associated medical morbidities. This intervention along with the support of appropriate technology and social environment is needed to maximize their quality of life and reduce dependency.

REHABILITATION RESOURCES IN MALAYSIA

Rehabilitation resources can be categorized as availability of human resources and health care providers (both public and private), educational and vocational, employment, sports, and information.

Over the years, more and more comprehensive and targeted information is being made available from government ministry Web sites related to disabilities (such as the Welfare Ministry, Ministry of Women and Children, Transport Ministry, MOH) as well as other locally initiated Web sites.[10,11]

From the rehabilitation health care provision point of view, active rehabilitation services are provided by governmental organizations and NGOs.

The government initiatives generally span across general hospitals, university hospitals, primary health, community-based rehabilitation centers, special schools, and welfare organizations (see **Table 2**).[10–13]

These institutions and organizations, however, do not always individually provide the full spectrum of rehabilitation services, but attempts have been made to ensure all states have reasonable facilities (**Table 1**).[10–12]

The rehabilitation services, although provided mainly by government hospitals under the MOH, have also worked with academic institutions under the Ministry of Higher Education to provide additional and tertiary level rehabilitation services. The facilities available in some of the smaller government hospitals are basic, unlike those in tertiary hospitals, which have more advanced technologies and therapies.

However, not all tertiary hospitals have a complete and comprehensive rehabilitation service team headed by rehabilitation medicine physicians. Presently, there are only about 100 rehabilitation medicine specialists to an estimated 3 million disabled in the population. These specialists are serving in MOH, Ministry of Education, and private hospitals throughout the country. The ratio of rehabilitation physicians to persons with disability is significantly low in Malaysia.

Of note is the establishment of a dedicated advanced level, comprehensive rehabilitation facility, namely, the Rehabilitation Hospital in Cheras, Kuala Lumpur, which is another major achievement by MOH toward strengthening the rehabilitative services in Malaysia. This Rehabilitation Hospital serves as the national referral center. The hospital started its operation in July 2012 and provides both inpatient and outpatient services. There are 6 wards (pediatric, spinal cord injury, stroke/neurology, geriatric, amputee/orthopedic, and traumatic brain injury/neurosurgery). Technologically advanced equipment is used for assessment, diagnosis, and treatment of the patients receiving care. Rehabilitation physician–led multidisciplinary approach is a key to handling every case to ensure a comprehensive and holistic care of the highest quality is provided to those in need.

COMMUNITY-BASED REHABILITATION CENTERS

The WHO has proposed the community-based rehabilitation model (CBR) as an appropriate model for developing countries to provide basic rehabilitation services to its citizens. In Malaysia, to date, there are hundreds of CBR centers all over Malaysia. They are mainly government funded. Klang Valley and Selangor areas alone have more than 60 CBR centers, which provide daycare rehabilitation services with the help of allied health personnel (**Table 2**).

During last few decades, the numbers of CBR centers have increased in urban areas, but accessibility to rehabilitation services and facilities is still limited in remote areas.

SPECIAL EDUCATION

The overall reported percentage of children with disabilities within the total student population in the national school system is inordinately low, at around 1%.[13] This amount could be due to limited accessible transport to school, inadequate facilities

Table 1
Overview of organizations providing rehabilitation facilities in various states of Malaysia

	Selangor & KL	Negeri Sembilan	Melaka	Johor	Perak	Pahang	Terengganu	Kelantan	Perlis	Pulau Pinang	Kedah	Sarawak	Sabah & Labuan	Total
Government	127	104	50	163	132	128	99	92	23	72	104	271	137	1502
NGO	219	35	28	77	79	14	7	6	4	65	17	40	36	626
Private	139	35	32	65	99	21	11	17	8	98	53	48	60	686
Miscellaneous	19	19	19	19	19	19	19	19	19	19	19	19	19	247

Table 2
Government-run facilities that provide rehabilitation services

	Number
Hospitals	136
Teaching hospitals	6
Primary health clinics	794
CBR	511
Special school	35
Social welfare services	16
Vocational training/workshops	4
Total	1502

and barrier-free environment within the national schools, and possibly some influence of social and cultural stigmata of disability.

There are 3 different schooling options provided by the Ministry of Education for children with disabilities under the national special needs education system.

a. Special education schools, which are specific schools for children with disabilities. There are currently 28 primary-level and 5 secondary-level special education schools. Of the 28 primary schools, 22 are for hearing impaired, 5 are for visually impaired, and 1 is for children with learning disabilities. Of the 5 secondary schools, 3 are vocational schools, while the remaining 2 are for the hearing impaired and the visually impaired, respectively.
b. Special education integrated programs (SEIP), which are specific classes in mainstream schools dedicated to children with special needs. There are currently just less than 2000 mainstream schools with SEIP, of which around 1300 are primary-level schools and around 670 are secondary-level schools.
c. Inclusive education programs, where children with disabilities are integrated into mainstream classes.

It is worth noting that the government has recognized that the inclusion of children with disabilities within mainstream schools through inclusive education programs is the most effective means of overcoming discriminatory attitudes and building an inclusive society and is in line with the government's commitment under the PWD Act to facilitate their "full and equal participation" in education.[13,14]

The Ministry of Education, through the Special Education Department, will need to work more with NGOs and the private education providers to strengthen the collaboration of social resources and work together in activities of training, seminars, outreach programs, smart partnerships, and inclusive programs to benefit children with the various disabilities.

The relevant ministries working together with NGO have also helped to establish vocational training centers and sporting facilities for people with disabilities. The NGOs also play a major role in advocacy and information resource for PWDs.[10-12]

THE PRIVATE SECTOR

The private sector functions mainly for profit but nonetheless helps fill the gaps in some areas of rehabilitation that are less available in government hospitals, like prosthetics and orthotics, specialized wheelchairs, and rehabilitation mobility devices.

They also help to serve communities that cannot afford the care, thereby helping to reduce traffic in the already congested government health facilities.

The services available in the private sector are private hospital services, private rehabilitation or stand-alone therapy services, nursing homes, equipment companies dealing with sale of medical and rehabilitation equipments, and even a few alternative therapies (**Table 3**).[11]

Unfortunately, many of the rehabilitation services provided by the private hospitals in Malaysia do not have the comprehensive rehabilitation and mainly are led by allied health personnel.

NONGOVERNMENTAL ORGANIZATIONS

As for the NGOs, fortunately most have diversified their efforts into forming organizations to address problems faced by the widely variable presentations of disabilities in adult and pediatric populations. These organizations are multifaceted in their function and form, ranging from providing limited to more specialized rehabilitation care, education, vocational, advocacy, funding, and information. Many faith-based organizations also make significant contributions to the above.

There are more than 200 NGOs centers concentrated in the central states of Selangor and Wilayah, which are the more developed states in West Malaysia (**Table 4**).[11]

RECOMMENDATIONS AND FUTURE DIRECTION

Based on the nation's need, the following can be recommended:

1. Safeguard rights of people living with disability.
2. Active involvement of more academic institutions in recruiting and training rehabilitation medicine trainees and offering fellowship training opportunities for subspecialties.
3. Development and implementation of an insurance health care coverage/funding policies for PWD.
4. Organized registry system for PWD as well as rehabilitation resources and workforces.
5. Awareness-raising seminars and workshops on disability and rehabilitation for public/community to encourage community engagement.
6. Outreach program/CBR to expand the coverage to far remote areas with poor rehabilitation services and facilities.
7. Training of more community disability workers, who can assist with health care services.

Table 3
Private centers that provide some rehabilitation services

	Number
Hospital	82
Nursing home with rehabilitation facilities	111
Rehabilitation centers	130
Medical equipment	96
Alternative therapies	267
Total	686

Table 4
Nongovernment organizations that provide limited rehabilitation services

	Number
Disabilities, adult	102
Disabilities, pediatrics	103
Faith	190
Health	148
Advocacy/funding/information	83
Total	626

SUMMARY

Rehabilitation service provision and capacity building have come a long way in Malaysia. Although it appears that Malaysia has a tremendous amount of rehabilitation support based on the centers and organizations available, more can be done to improve service delivery. There is also a need for these services to reach the rural population. The current system is still fragmented, with little collaboration. A structured, workable model is needed, which should be part of an integrated and coordinated system with strategic plans that take into account the ever-changing needs of PWDs.

ACKNOWLEDGMENTS

The authors thank the following for assistance rendered in preparation of this article: Dr Manimalar Selvi Naicker (MBBS, MPath, MMed Stats), lecturer and consultant, University Malaya, Malaysia; Ang Chun Yiing, Medical graduate, International Medical University, Kuala Lumpur, Malaysia; Edwin Sam Keat Song, Medical graduate, International Medical University, Kuala Lumpur, Malaysia.

REFERENCES

1. Laws of Malaysia. Online version of updated text of reprint. Persons with Disabilities Act 2008. Available at: https://www.ilo.org/dyn/natlex/docs/ELECTRONIC/86297/117930/F139356912/MYS86297.pdf. Accessed November 25, 2018.
2. Convention on the Rights of Persons with Disabilities (CRPD). Available at: https://www.un.org/development/desa/disabilities/convention-on-the-rights-of-persons-with-disabilities.html. Accessed November 25, 2018.
3. Population distribution and basic demographic characteristic report 2010. Department of Statistics Malaysia; 2011. Official Portal of Department of Statistics Malaysia; Released 2011. Available at: https://www.dosm.gov.my/. Accessed August 14, 2019.
4. Online registration for disability in Malaysia. Available at: http://oku.jkm.gov.my/smoku_online.html. Accessed November 25, 2018.
5. Official portal of Dept of Social Welfare, Malaysia. Available at: http://www.jkm.gov.my/. Accessed November 25, 2018.
6. Ahmad NA, Mohamad Kasim N, Mahmud NA, et al. Prevalence and determinants of disability among adults in Malaysia: results from the National Health and Morbidity Survey (NHMS) 2015. BMC Public Health 2017;17(1):756.
7. United Nations regional meeting on disability measurement and statistics in support of the 2030 agenda for sustainable development and the 2020 world population and housing census programme. Malaysian experience.

Available at: https://unstats.un.org/unsd/demographic-social/meetings/2016/
bangkok–disability-measurement-and-statistics/Session-6/Malaysia.pdf. Accessed
November 20, 2018.

8. Health care program for person with disabilities, plan of action 2011-2020. Book
Publication by Family Health Development Division, Public Health Department,
Ministry of health Malaysia; 2011.

9. Global Disability Plan of Action, Family Health Development Division, Public
Health Department, Ministry of Health Malaysia.

10. Available at: https://www.malaysia.gov.my. Accessed November 20, 2018.

11. Available at: https://mind.org.my/. Accessed November 20, 2018.

12. Available at: http://www.malaysiancare.org/directories-resources/. Accessed
November 20, 2018.

13. Malaysian education blueprint 2013 - 2025 . Book published by Ministry of Education Malaysia, 2013. Chapter 4. p. 4–17.

14. Unicef 2013: Children with disabilities in Malaysia Mapping the Policies, Programmes, Interventions and Stakeholders. Prepared by Mahaletchumi Balak-
rishnan and Vizla Kumaresan Produced by child protection section of Unicef
Malaysia, 2014.

Rehabilitation in South India

Raji Thomas, MBBS, DPMR, MD(PMR), DNB(PMR)*,
George Tharion, MBBS, DPMR, D Ortho, DNB(PMR), MD(PMR)

KEYWORDS

- Spinal cord injury • Brain injury • Rehabilitation research

KEY POINTS

- The article describes the rehabilitation services provided at Christian Medical College Vellore, a tertiary care medical college hospital in South India.
- The department was started by Dr Mary Verghese, who on completion of her medical training sustained spinal cord injury and paraplegia.
- Comprehensive rehabilitation is provided to patients with disabling conditions coming from all over the country.
- The department has been designated as a World Health Organization Collaborating Center.
- The article ends with challenges faced, including financial limitations, architectural and attitudinal barriers, and inadequate number of rehabilitation physicians and comprehensive rehabilitation centers in the country.

DESTINY OR DESIGN?

The Department of Physical Medicine and Rehabilitation was set up at Christian Medical College (CMC), Vellore, India, in 1964 by Dr Mary Verghese[1] (**Fig. 1**). CMC Vellore is a 2500-bedded tertiary care medical college hospital in South India established in 1900. Dr Verghese was a young medical graduate from CMC with dreams of becoming an obstetrician, following the footsteps of Dr Ida Scudder, an American doctor who founded the institution. Unfortunately, Dr Verghese was involved in a major road traffic accident in 1954. She survived the road crash but suffered spinal cord injury that left her paraplegic. Dreams shattered, she considered that she would not be of any use in the medical field. Fortunately, Dr Paul

Disclosure Statement: The authors have nothing to disclose.
Department of Physical Medicine and Rehabilitation, Christian Medical College Vellore, Vellore, Tamil Nadu, India
* Corresponding author.
E-mail address: rajithomas@cmcvellore.ac.in

Phys Med Rehabil Clin N Am 30 (2019) 817–833
https://doi.org/10.1016/j.pmr.2019.07.011

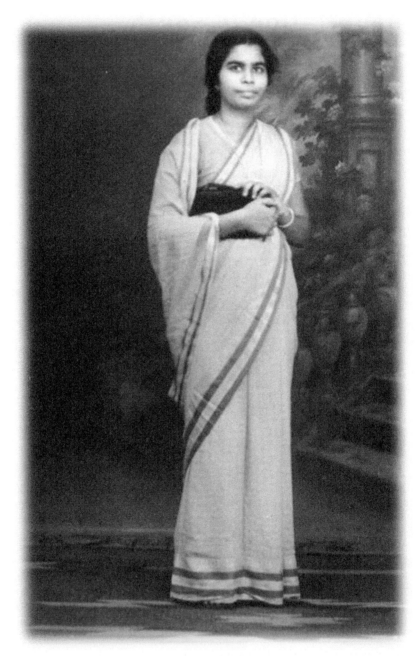

Fig. 1. Dr Mary Verghese.

Brand, a pioneer orthopedic surgeon at CMC Vellore had already started his groundbreaking work in the surgical reconstruction and rehabilitation of hand deformities in patients with leprosy. Dr Brand inspired Dr Varghese to take on a new challenge to be a surgeon from the wheelchair.[1]

In 1957, Dr Varghese went to Australia where she completed her own rehabilitation, learned wheelchair skills, and achieved functional independence under the care of Sir George Bedbrook at the Royal Perth Hospital in Australia. She now realized that patients in India who were similarly afflicted did not have an avenue for rehabilitation following such disabling conditions. She took on this challenge and moved to New York on a fellowship obtained through the World Rehabilitation Fund to complete the Diplomate of the American Board of Physical Medicine and Rehabilitation under Professor Howard Rusk, Director of the Institute of Rehabilitation, New York[1] (**Fig. 2**).

On her return in 1964, she started the Department of Physical Medicine and Rehabilitation in Vellore, which was inaugurated by then-President of India, Dr S. Radhakrishnan. Dr Varghese's new ventures received attention, and patients with spinal injuries from all over the country began traveling to Vellore for their rehabilitation.

On November 26, 1966, Dr Verghese started a specially designed Rehabilitation Institute located 7 km from the main hospital.[1] Here, patients could be admitted for a few months of rehabilitation (**Fig. 3**) to learn independence, practice mobility skills, and acquire vocational skills to survive in the community. Patients with spinal cord injuries saw a glimmer of light in their lives, and Dr Verghese, popularly known as the Wheelchair Surgeon, held the torch high as a beacon to guide and assist in their difficult journeys.

Dr Verghese envisioned that excellent teamwork is crucial for an efficient rehabilitation. She started services and education in physiotherapy, occupational therapy, and prosthetic and orthotic services. Social integration and exploration of vocational opportunities were facilitated by the social workers who worked closely with the team. She initiated home visits and sports for disabled individuals (**Fig. 4**), and started the electrodiagnostic laboratory to study peripheral nerve disorders.[2]

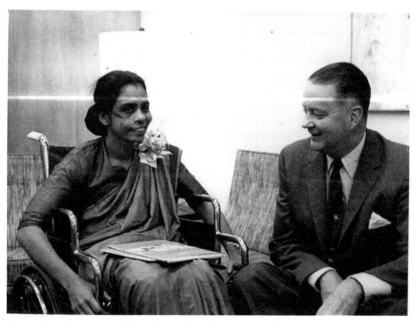

Fig. 2. Dr Mary Verghese with Dr Howard Rusk in New York.

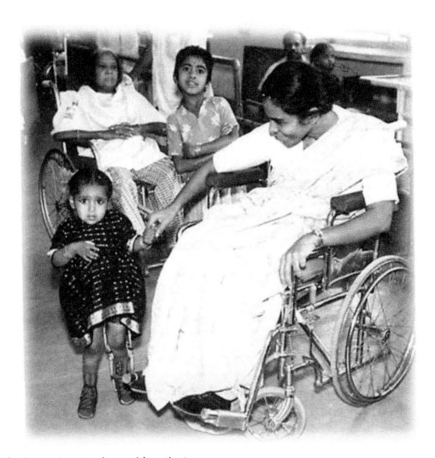

Fig. 3. Dr Mary Verghese with patients.

In 1972, the nation honored Dr Varghese with Padmashri, one of the highest civilian awards in the country, for her pioneering work, which she did with courage, fortitude, and indomitable enthusiasm (**Fig. 5**).

The work that she began continued in congruence with her vision. In 2016, the department celebrated 50 years of relentless service. By then, the growth has been steady and encouraging, attending to larger number of patients, offering a wider spectrum of rehabilitation services and contributing to postgraduate education and research in accordance with the mission statement of the institution.

CLINICAL SERVICES

Currently the department has the capacity to accommodate 150 inpatients. Approximately 800 patients are admitted and 22,500 patients are seen in the outpatient section annually. The medical team has 24 doctors and there is a large multidisciplinary team of physiotherapists, occupational therapists, speech therapists, prosthetists and orthotists, social workers, nurses, psychologists, rehabilitation engineers, and related professionals. It was soon recognized that patients with other severe disabilities following brain injury, stroke, and cerebral palsy were languishing

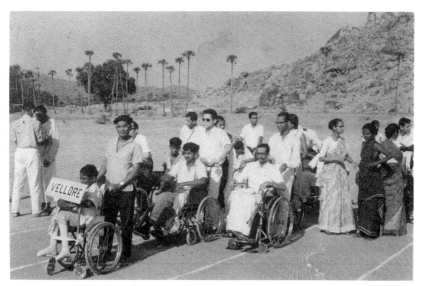

Fig. 4. Sports for the disabled.

without rehabilitation and needed attention. In response to this need, services were extended to address the needs of these patients.

ACUTE MANAGEMENT

Patients travel thousands of miles seeking help, due to dearth of comprehensive rehabilitation facilities elsewhere in the country. The acute ward admits patients from the outpatient section, emergency services, or on referral from other specialties. Medical complications such as pneumonia, seizures, and thromboembolism, are managed. Pressure sores are a major preventable complication. Several patients may have already developed pressure sores at the time of their admission. They are managed conservatively or surgically with skin grafts and fasciocutaneous flaps as necessary. Some patients present with infected hips needing hip excision to save them from life threatening septicemia. All efforts are taken to prevent pressure sores, including education of patients and family by the team. Commercially available cushions are beyond the financial reach of most patients, and hence a low-cost cushion has been developed as an alternative, with an air pillow at the rear and foam block in the front, which by now, has stood the test of time. Other surgeries, including multiple soft tissue release, cystolitholapaxy, and suprapubic cystostomy are performed once a week by the rehabilitation physicians.

REHABILITATION

Once management in the acute ward is over, patients continue their treatment at the Rehabilitation Institute, where they spend 2 to 3 months for their physical, psychological, and social rehabilitation along with their immediate family members. Here patients are assessed by the various team members, following which an initial meeting is conducted to decide goals, outcome, timeline, and logistics of rehabilitation. Progress is evaluated by the team periodically every week and at midterm. A predischarge evaluation is done to assess if the goals have been accomplished as planned. The patient

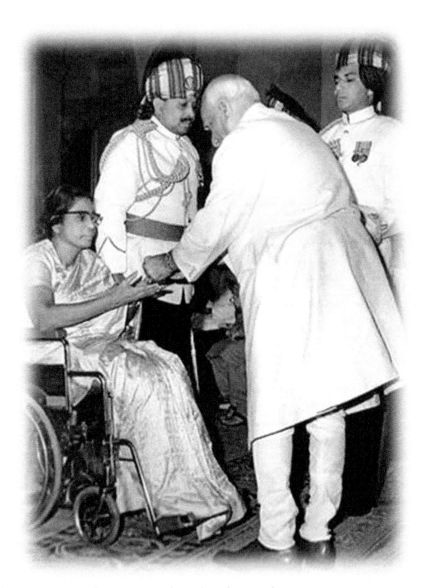

Fig. 5. Dr Mary Verghese receiving the Padma Shri award.

and family take active participation in the decision making process, expressing their fears, goals, and aspirations as they form an integral part of the rehabilitation team. These meetings help to formulate realistic, time-bound goals and integrated interventions to achieve the best possible outcome for the patient. The focus is always on the patient and family, empowering the family to look after the patient.

"Will I be able to walk" is the first question asked by most of our patients. Hence, restoring mobility is the primary concern. Patients are mobilized initially on a prone trolley with wheels and push rim which encourages them to propel independently. Although the wheelchair is an energy-efficient method of ambulation, in developing

countries like India, wheelchair users encounter insurmountable architectural barriers limiting their mobility, as well as social and vocational opportunities. These constraints predispose the wheelchair users to more complications than those who are ambulant with other orthotic devices. Hence, intense efforts are undertaken to mobilize patients using lightweight orthotic appliances as permitted by the residual neurologic function and comorbidities.

In case of spinal cord injuries, patients with neurologic level T10 and below are trained to walk with the help of knee ankle foot orthosis and elbow crutches. Advanced training helps them to walk on rough terrain as well as to negotiate ramps and stairs so that they regain confidence to reintegrate into the community.

With higher neurological levels, wheelchair independence is set as the goal, and for tetraplegic patients with limited upper limb function, motorized wheelchair training is provided. Independence is facilitated by training in activities of daily living, transfers, and prevocational skills. Appropriate assistive devices and compensatory strategies are instituted as required. Patients are taken to the community on completion of training to instill confidence in carrying out day to day errands.

Pursuit of lightweight materials for orthotic fabrication opened up research opportunities with the Fiber Reinforced Plastic Center at IIT Madras, Chennai. This joint endeavor was supported by the Department of Science and Technology, Government of India. This led to the setting up of the gait analysis laboratory in 1989 (**Fig. 6**), making it possible to measure the efficiency of ambulation[3] using different orthotic appliances of varying weights and designs. Coordinated work with the rehabilitation engineering team helps to explore optimal solutions to complex problems. The International Committee of the Red Cross (ICRC) supported the efforts to integrate lightweight materials, such as polypropylene, in the fabrication of orthosis and prosthesis, and this paradigm shift in strategy made these appliances lighter, modular, weather resistant, and mechanically advantageous. It enabled the appliances to be fabricated in a shorter time. Further, due to the thermoplastic properties of these materials, the devices could be modified even after the completion of fabrication. A low-cost electrical upper limb prosthesis was fabricated in 2003.

Spasticity is a major concern during training for mobility and functional independence. Most often it is addressed with incremental dosages of baclofen, tizanidine, or benzodiazepines. Focal spasticity is managed with local injection of botulinum toxin under ultrasound image guidance. Peripheral nerve blocks[4] with electromyography guidance are administered as appropriate. Intrathecal baclofen pump is inserted for disabling spasticity that is not amenable to conventional strategies.

Neurogenic bladder is another perpetual concern of patients with neurologic illnesses. Indian Council Medical Research (ICMR) supported exploring low-cost

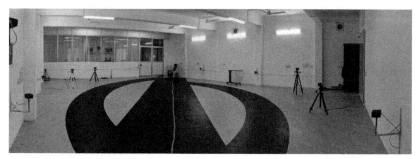

Fig. 6. Gait analysis laboratory.

options to address this distressing symptom.[5] Evaluation using urodynamic studies, cystoscopy, and ultrasonographic imaging to determine the best course of management of neurogenic bladder soon became the standard of care. Patients are taught self-intermittent clean catheterization when hand functions are adequate. Detrusor hyperreflexia is managed with anticholinergics, and in occasional cases, botulinum toxin is injected into the bladder. Incontinence resulting from an open bladder neck has been more difficult to manage, and a trial of sympathomimetic medications is offered with partial success. Suprapubic catheterization has been found to be a better option for patients with tetraplegia. Recent research on tibial nerve stimulation to reduce detrusor hyperreflexia demonstrated its effectiveness and has led to further studies as a nonpharmacologic alternative.[6] A low-cost CMG machine is also being developed. As part of sexual rehabilitation, family counselling, systemic or topical agents to assist sexual functions, as well as vibrector-assisted ejaculation for fertility, is offered wherever indicated.

Patients with acquired brain injury have more complex deficits, affecting their language, speech, and cognition. As part of cognitive retraining, strategies to compensate for deficits in memory, attention, planning, judgment, and visuospatial problems are explored. Speech therapists strive to improve speech and communication as well as to ensure safe swallowing. Patients with severe difficulties in language are evaluated for the usefulness of alternate and augmentative communication aids. Environmental control devices are given when appropriate. Psychologists address various neurobehavioral and cognitive issues, and provides counselling to patients and their families to overcome the period of denial and grief. In addition, there is regular input from the psychiatry team.

A specially dedicated pediatric rehabilitation service was set up in 2011, recognizing the need to treat young children in a holistic and child-friendly manner. Families are given guidance regarding preschool skills, educational opportunities, and training for life skills.

COMMUNITY REINTEGRATION

Many patients come to rehabilitation after a life-altering situation, raising questions, doubts, and fears that are beyond human understanding. The chapel at the heart of Rehabilitation Institute provide strength and spiritual solace to many. Group therapy sessions are an avenue for patients to ventilate their anxieties and apprehensions. Peer interaction is an invaluable resource for coping enabling patients to have realistic expectations. The importance of being independent and having a vocation are emphasized. Picnics, celebration of national days and festivals as well as art therapy sessions instil courage and confidence in patients for community reintegration.

SPORTS

Sports games, are encouraged during the rehabilitation process which improves self-esteem and dignity. Several rehabilitated patients have represented the country in wheelchair basketball competition and had spectacular success at the national level (**Fig. 7**).

HOME VISITS

Social workers link the patient and family with the community. They do an initial home visit while the patient is in the hospital to explore the local resources, support systems, and environmental accessibility so that contextually appropriate goals can be made.

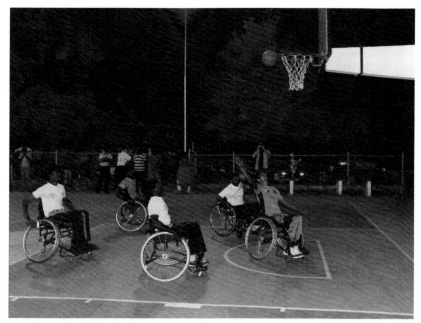

Fig. 7. Wheelchair basketball.

They assist the patient and families to cope with various challenges arising from disability and give guidance regarding future vocational opportunities. In addition, they educate patients regarding their rights, responsibilities and social security benefits.

VOCATIONAL TRAINING

In 1993, a vocational rehabilitation project for the severely disabled persons was initiated. Various vocations, including tailoring, bicycle repair, basket weaving, and cane work, which are likely to sustain in the rural villages have been explored (**Fig. 8**). Following inpatient rehabilitation, suitable patients are provided training for 6 months to learn these skills. This empowers them to earn social identity and contribute meaningfully to families and communities. A survey among patients who have been trained showed that 92% were continuing to practice their vocation.

FOLLOW-UP

Patients and relatives return home on completion of the rehabilitation and must survive on their own where they have to battle architectural and attitudinal barriers with economic constraints. Maintaining links to the Rehabilitation Center was found to be crucial to sustain the spirit and enthusiasm of patients with disabilities. However, patients find it difficult to navigate the long queues and access institutional rehabilitation services. To overcome this, various follow-up strategies, including review home visits, support groups, and annual review fairs, have been set up.[7] The multidisciplinary team from the department routinely undertakes monthly home visits to these villages covering the follow-up area up to 100 km (**Fig. 9**). This helps to foster links as well as address simple problems and explore locally relevant solutions. A database

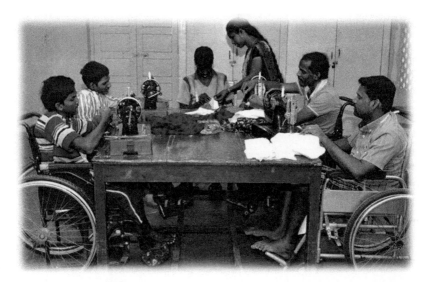

Fig. 8. Vocational training.

of nearly 1000 rehabilitated patients is maintained and monitored by the GPS system.

Monthly support groups provide social and recreational activities and guidance on coping strategies, and provide an avenue for medical follow-up (**Fig. 10**). Further, once a year all patients and their families gather for their medical review, which has been organized since 1994 in the form of a festival popularly known as the Rehab Mela (Fair) (**Fig. 11**). This provides an opportunity for patients to be reassessed by the rehabilitation physician and the treating team; to conduct blood tests, ultrasound imaging, cystoscopic evaluation, and to avail any necessary services. This also serves as an opportunity for peer counseling, as patients derive enrichment from each other's life experiences. Following medical evaluation, patients engage in sports, competitions, talent shows, group sessions, and spiritual discussions. The event ends with discussion of the medical reports with the patients. A separate Brain Injury Mela was initiated in 2004. Regional melas are organized for patients who are unable to participate for various reasons, and our team offers support to conduct these events.

COMMUNITY-BASED REHABILITATION

It was soon realized that the Rehabilitation Institute with all its efforts would not be able to meet the needs of a vast number of disabled people in the community. To address these lacunae, community-based rehabilitation (CBR) was launched, along with a Low-Cost Effective Care Unit of the Community Health Department. This venture was supported by the World Health Organization (WHO), which was exploring a sustainable model of CBR that could survive in a developing country like India. CBR was initiated among a local population of 20,000 in Vellore, located at an economically disadvantaged and impoverished part of this town (**Fig. 12**). Volunteers are recruited and trained using WHO training modules to identify problems and propose solutions that were locally relevant using limited resources in consultation with the team from the secondary and tertiary centers. Such need-based approach is welcomed by the

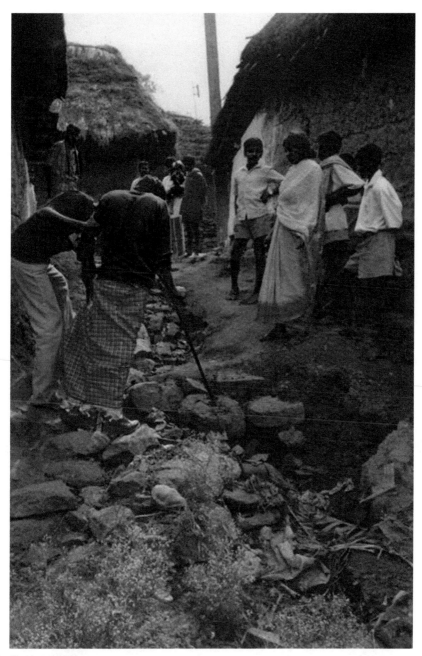

Fig. 9. Home visits.

community as well. These initial efforts with CBR subsequently opened up other in-roads into the community, leading to many other satellite initiatives including a school education program (**Fig. 13**), injury prevention program, elderly rehabilitation program, and life skill training program for the youth in the community.

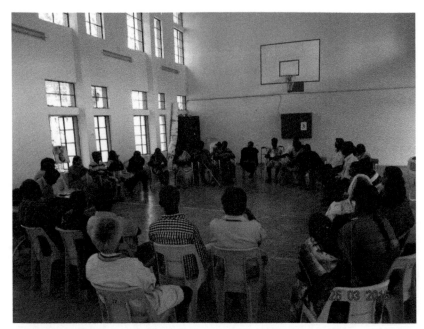

Fig. 10. Support groups.

OUTPATIENT SERVICES

The outpatient service of the department attends to patients who are ambulant, which includes those with musculoskeletal problems, chronic pain, neuromuscular disorders, diabetic foot, amputations, and sequel of spinal cord and acquired brain injuries. The hemophilia clinic helps patients with arthropathy and multiple joint deformities following recurrent bleeds. Prophylactic factor replacement is not an option due

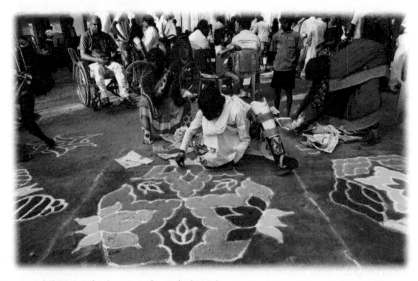

Fig. 11. Exhibition of talents at the Rehab Mela.

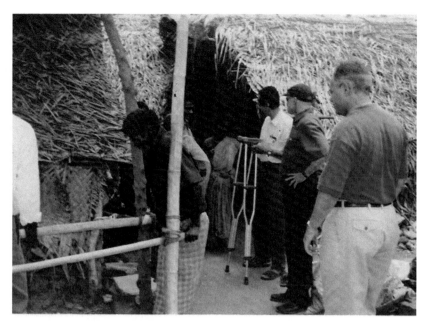

Fig. 12. Community-based rehabilitation.

to the exorbitant costs and hence many patients present with severe deformities of the knees and elbows due to joint and muscle bleeds.[8,9] Exercises, serial plaster casting, splinting, and surgery are done to correct these contractures. Radiosynoviorthesis with Yttrium is done for synovitis in coordination with the Hematology and Nuclear Medicine departments. The Neuromuscular Clinic evaluates patients with muscular dystrophies, myopathies, and anterior horn cell diseases along with the departments of Neurology and Clinical Genetics. Electrodiagnostic evaluation of peripheral nerve injuries is routinely performed in the department[10]

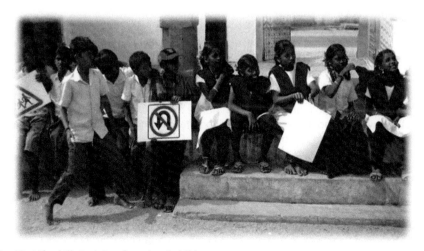

Fig. 13. Life skills training for school children.

EDUCATION

Educating new graduates and disseminating the knowledge and skills is of utmost importance because there is dearth of good rehabilitation services and centers across this country. This is in resonance to the mission of the CMC, which strives to develop compassionate, professionally excellent, and ethically sound professionals. The department conducts several educational courses, such as MD in Physical Medicine and Rehabilitation for medical graduates, graduate and postgraduate courses in physiotherapy, graduate courses in occupational therapy and prosthetic and orthotic services. Rehabilitation Medicine has been included in the medical undergraduate curriculum and is a part of the compulsory rotatory internship. This has helped to improve awareness regarding the spread and scope of the specialty.

RESEARCH

Research is given an important thrust in the department. Currently, research activities are conducted in a spectrum of subjects related to rehabilitation. Facilities like Gait Laboratory, Urodynamic Laboratory, Cell Culture Laboratory, Prosthetic and Orthotic Facility, and CBR also widen the scope of research. Research has been supported by the Government of India through the Department of Science and Technology (DST), Department of Biotechnology (DBT), Indian Council of Medical Research (ICMR), International Committee of Red Cross (ICRC), Christopher Blinden Mission, and WHO, as well as funds from within the institution. By the dawn of this century, reports of stem cell transplantation possibly improving neurologic outcome in patients with spinal cord injury started emerging. A in-depth study in this regard was initiated. A laboratory for spinal cord regeneration research was set up with the support of DBT, Goverment of India for this purpose. Experiments were conducted to explore the benefits of transplantation of cells like olfactory ensheathing cells and bone marrow stromal cells, and also the effect of agents like chondroitinase and local growth factors in rat models of spinal cord injury.[11,12]

WORLD HEALTH ORGANIZATION COLLABORATING CENTER

In recognition of the wide range of activities being conducted, the department has been designated as a WHO Collaborating Center for Development of Rehabilitation Technology, Capacity Building, and Disability Prevention. Guidelines were prepared for the care of patients with spinal cord injury in the community. WHO fellows from North Korea, Myanmar, and Sri Lanka have regularly received training in various disciplines related to rehabilitation.

CHALLENGES

While center is trying to reach out to alleviate the burden of disability, there are several challenges which need to be confronted concurrently. Scarcity of funds to meet medical expenditures continues to haunt the system. Often it is the sole earning member of the family who falls victim to these disabling life-changing events, which not only drains the existing resources, but also stops any further earning. The mission of the institution is to reach out to the marginalized and the economically disadvantaged and although it has instituted several avenues to alleviate this burden by offering concessional services. However, the financial need far outweighs the available resources. These constraints compel the team to be innovative and creative, and to devise low-cost solutions wherever possible. Thus, providing affordable services continues to be a challenge.

Early resuscitation and enhanced intensive care services have facilitated the survival of patients who otherwise would have succumbed to their increasingly severe disabling conditions. This raises a new challenge of patients requiring advanced rehabilitative interventions, such as robotic-assisted aids, environmental control systems, specially equipped wheel chairs, augmentative communicative systems, bionic hands, virtual reality training, and brain computer interface systems. However, these expensive solutions are beyond the reach of most patients who will benefit from them.

Further, architectural barriers that patients must overcome, be it at home, in the community, work place, or public transport systems curtail their independence (**Fig. 14**). Most houses are not barrier free and the scope to modify them is limited by the nonexistence of funds or support systems to address these barriers. Community rehabilitation services are almost not available in most parts of the country and hence patients are confined to their homes. Attitudinal barriers with the social stigma associated with the disability are not uncommon. The rehabilitation follow-up services available in the community are limited and therefore patients have to resort to tertiary hospital services when required.

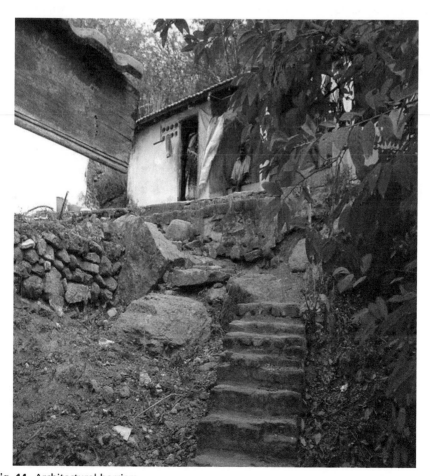

Fig. 14. Architectural barriers.

Universally the emphasis for rehabilitation is inadequate, and this reflects in the Indian context as well. Preventive and curative medicine rightfully has a major share, whereas rehabilitation services often suffer from resource crunch and lack of professionals to work as an integrated team. Currently postgraduate training in Physical Medicine and Rehabilitation is offered in different parts of the country. Moreover, several allied health training centers are also available across India. But for a population of more than 1 billion, the number of specialists and rehabilitation services available is grossly inadequate. Hence, patients who need rehabilitation after the acute event continue to languish in hospitals and homes while waiting for an opportunity to get access to rehabilitation services and restore their lives. In the meantime, they develop preventable complications like pressure sores, contractures, and heterotopic ossification, which further add on to the expenses, complexity, duration, and ultimate outcome of rehabilitation.

Physical Medicine and Rehabilitation in South India has made steady impressive progress over the past few decades. It has miles to go, but still has endured a difficult voyage and it is heartening to note that awareness of the need for rehabilitation among professionals and patients is on the rise, with more young and enthusiastic professionals joining the field. It is envisaged that in the near future there will be specialized regional rehabilitation centers of excellence in all major cities with peripheral satellite rehabilitation facilities in the district and community levels in India, making rehabilitative care available and accessible to all.

REFERENCES

1. Take My Hands-The Remarkable Story of Dr Mary Verghese of Vellore; Dorothy Clarke Wilson.
2. Verghese M, Radhakrishnan M, Chandrapal H, et al. Phasic conversion after tibialis posterior transfer. Arch Phys Med Rehabil 1975;56(2):83–5.
3. Thomas R, Ganesh T, George J, et al. Instrumented gait analysis for planning and assessment of treatment in cerebral palsy. Indian J Orthop 2005;39(3):182.
4. Rajendra K, Venugopal K, George T, et al. A study to evaluate the effectiveness of Phenol blocks to peripheral nerves in reducing spasticity in patients with paraplegia and brain injury. Indian Journal of Physical Medicine & Rehabilitation 2008;19(1):13–7.
5. George J, Tharion G, Richard J, et al. The effectiveness of intravesical oxybutynin, propantheline, and capsaicin in the management of neuropathic bladder following spinal cord injury. ScientificWorldJournal 2007;7:1683–90.
6. Ojha R, George J, Chandy BR, et al. Neuromodulation by surface electrical stimulation of peripheral nerves for reduction of detrusor overactivity in patients with spinal cord injury: a pilot study. J Spinal Cord Med 2015;38(2):207–13.
7. Barman A, Shanmugasundaram D, Bhide R, et al. Survival in persons with traumatic spinal cord injury receiving structured follow-up in South India. Arch Phys Med Rehabil 2014;95(4):642–8.
8. John JA, Mani RM, Thomas R, et al. Low-cost treatment for haemophilic knee contractures. BMJ Rapid responses 6 April 2007 to Editorial by Christine Lee, Caroline Sabin, and Alexander Miners. High cost, low volume care: the case of haemophilia. BMJ 1997;315:962–3.
9. Fischer K, Van den Berg HM, Thomas R, et al. Dose and outcome of care in haemophilia–how do we define cost-effectiveness? Haemophilia 2004;10(Suppl 4): 216–20.

10. Barman A, Chatterjee A, Prakash H, et al. Traumatic brachial plexus injury: electrodiagnostic findings from 111 patients in a tertiary care hospital in India. Injury 2012;43(11):1943–8.
11. Sabapathy V, Tharion G, Kumar S. Cell therapy augments functional recovery subsequent to spinal cord injury under experimental conditions. Stem Cells Int 2015;2015:e132172.
12. Tharion G, Indrani K, Durai M, et al. Motor Recovery following olfactory ensheathing cell transplantation in rats with spinal cord injury. Neurology India 2011;59(4): 566–72.

Rehabilitation in Low-Resource Areas

Mrinal Joshi, MBBS, MD, DNB, MNAMS, GCMskMed

KEYWORDS

- Community-based rehabilitation (CBR) • Health-related rehabilitation
- Multipurpose rehabilitation worker • International classification of functioning (ICF)
- Telerehabilitation • Task-shifting • Disability

KEY POINTS

- The World Health Survey indicates that more than half of the people with disability were not able to afford health services in comparison to 30% of people without disabilities.
- Community-based rehabilitation (CBR) has established itself as a useful tool to address health-related rehabilitative services to people with disabilities in low-resource areas.
- The community should be ready to initiate, accept, develop, and implement CBR among themselves.
- Task shifting to an alternative cadre in resource-poor areas is a promising option to deliver health-related rehabilitation services.
- CBR should receive planning, guidance and training, and management inputs from physical medicine and rehabilitation specialists to truly integrate CBR in the health system.

INTRODUCTION

Disability is universal, and all of us are likely to experience it directly or indirectly through our family members at some point in life. According to the World Health Organization (WHO), 1 billion people are living with disabilities, that is 15% of the total population; most of them, 80%, are living in low- and middle-income countries.[1]

People with disabilities living in low- and middle-income countries are "without a voice," thus remain marginalized and disparaged socially. Despite the ongoing development in these countries, it remains challenging for them to access not only rehabilitative but also general health care services. It pushes them more toward poor health, economic poverty, and adverse living conditions.

Poverty and disability have a causal nexus, and failure to address disability issues will lead to unattainable Sustainable Development Goals (SDG), and the health and

Disclosure Statement: The author has nothing to disclose.
Department of Physical Medicine and Rehabilitation, Rehabilitation Research Center, SMS Medical College & Hospital, Sawai Jai Singh Road, Jaipur 302004, India
E-mail address: dr.m.joshi@gmail.com

Phys Med Rehabil Clin N Am 30 (2019) 835–846
https://doi.org/10.1016/j.pmr.2019.07.007
pmr.theclinics.com

social impacts of failing to receive necessary rehabilitation services will affect greatly those who are already the most disadvantaged economically.[2]

The World Health Surveys indicate that more than half of people with disabilities were unable to afford health services in comparison to 30% of people without disabilities. The WHO's Global Disability Action Plan thus pushes to increase access to rehabilitation as well as health services among people with disabilities.[3]

There is also an epidemiologic and demographic change happening whereby the trend is shifting toward higher prevalence of chronic and noncommunicable disease, an increase by 13.7% in the past 10 years according to Global Burden of Disease (2015). For the increasing aging population, long-term care and rehabilitation will be necessary. Chronic diseases now account for almost 66.5% of all years lived with disability in low-income and middle-income countries.

The WHO Disability Action Plan (2014–2021) has the following 3 objectives[4]: Removing barriers and improving access to health services and programs; strengthening and extending rehabilitation, habilitation, assistive technology, assistance, and support services, and community-based rehabilitation (CBR); and improving the collection of relevant and comparable data on disability to support research on disability and related services internationally.

It underscores the implementation of the United Nations (UN) convention on the Rights of Person with Disabilities, and WHO asserts the following components to build better health systems and services[5]:

- Health service delivery
- Health workforce
- Health information system
- Access to essential medicines
- Financing
- Leadership and governance

Despite the implementation of the UN Convention for the Rights of People with Disabilities, more than 40% of countries neither adopted rehabilitation policies nor programs, and also more than 50% of countries have not even passed any legislation on rehabilitation for people with disabilities.[6]

Universal Health Coverage states, "ensuring all people have access to the needed promotive, preventive, curative, rehabilitative, and palliative services they need, of sufficient quality to be effective while ensuring that the use of these services results in financial hardship". It is recognized as a critical earmark for SDGs and providing rehabilitation is essential to reach the SDGs. Access to rehabilitation services to the challenged person is also a human right, as stated in the UN Convention for the Rights of People with Disabilities.

REHABILITATION SERVICES DELIVERY IN A LOW-RESOURCE AREA

Most of the published research on models, place, and team approach to deliver rehabilitation services has occurred in high-income countries, and there is an urgent need for more evidence in resource-limited settings.[7]

In the last 4 decades, CBR has established itself as a useful tool to address health-related rehabilitative services, including health-related rehabilitation services to people with disabilities in low-resource areas. WHO has defined CBR as a strategy for rehabilitation, social inclusion, empowerment, economic development, and equalization of opportunities among the disabled.

During the early years, CBR was a medical model with emphasis on the individual, focused medical and surgical interventions, and therapy. The social model started in the western hemisphere during the 1970s, weighing more social activities for the inclusion of disabled in all aspects of society.[8]

In last few decades, it has been slowly been realized that the CBR centers, although excluding health-related rehabilitation services, have failed to achieve their goal because they got separated from the mainstream health services and remained isolated service models, particularly in low- and middle-income countries. Also, in poor societies wherein the bread winner has become disabled, there was a role change for other family members, making it difficult for them to attend the CBR group, whereby there was no health or health-related solutions for their problems, for example, advice for home modifications for a paraplegic in a rural area with limited resources.[8]

According to WHO, rehabilitation is a set of interventions designed to optimize functioning and reduce disability in individuals with health conditions in interaction with their environment. Therefore, from a health perspective, rehabilitation is one of the health strategies, that is, preventive, curative, rehabilitative, palliative, and supportive strategies. It is a part of the continuum care that can be delivered through a primary health center.

Currently, a comprehensive model is being promoted whereby the CBR should not only cover health and health-related rehabilitation but also include interventions focused on better education, livelihood, social inclusion, and empowerment at single point access as specified in the WHO CBR matrix. Gutenbrunner and his team strongly recommended that the rehabilitation programs should get institutionalized by aligning with preexisting ministerial models of health care in order to support program sustainability.[8,9]

CBR has evolved through time and has proven itself as a way to achieve a 360° rehabilitation intervention/development in low-resource areas, but also it must be understood that it does not and cannot replace secondary or tertiary level rehabilitation services. The WHO global disability action plan (2014–2021) makes it clear that both kinds of services are obligations of states as to the right of people with disabilities.[4,9]

There is moderate to high-quality evidence that a multidisciplinary, specialized rehabilitation unit should support acute and complex clients with later follow-up in outpatients, at the district level or in the community through CBR to reach the rehabilitation goals, and less complicated clients can continue to attend the multidisciplinary teams in hospital outpatient services or community/clinic settings.[7] Such integrated interventions will reduce the complications and enhance recovery and thereby reduce the burden on the family as well as on the health system. The social and vocational rehabilitation can initiate at any level of contact to provide early guidance to social inclusion, social benefit, and return to work. Moreover, a multidisciplinary team at the tertiary level can support the grass root multipurpose rehabilitation worker for follow-up at the community level, addressing problems that transpire. The integration of rehabilitation in the continuum care across all levels of health systems will help to achieve person-centered care.[10] The Guidelines Development Group also recommends that health-related rehabilitation should come under the ambit of the ministry of health because rehabilitation is a health strategy in conjunction with other health services using common resources.[11,12]

In 2004, the CBR matrix was proposed (**Fig. 1**) with 5 key components and variously related subheadings.[9] It gives an option to choose the most practical entry point depending on local needs and capacity. It will slowly be built up to form a strong alliance with different sectors until they are well established in society.

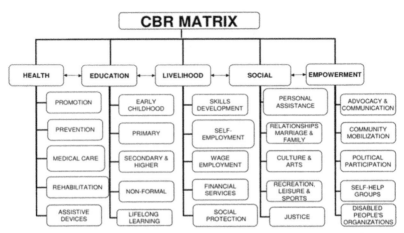

Fig. 1. CBR matrix. (*From* World Health Organization. CBR matrix. Available at: https://www. who.int/disabilities/cbr/cbr_matrix_11.10.pdf; with permission.)

CBR can be managed by the ministry of health while collaborating with social service providers, but the priorities can change from medical to social depending on the priority area. To improve penetration, to provide health and rehabilitation services, to strengthen referral services and long-term sustainability, and to save duplication of funds, it should integrate with primary health care centers (PHCs) at the village level. It will help to improve data collection on disability-causing diseases, provide health-related rehabilitation, and ascertain the quality of life among the clients who benefit. By integrating, it is recommended that health-related rehabilitation should be financed, managed, and promoted like any other general health service program as part of universal health coverage and SDG.[8]

COMMUNITY-BASED REHABILITATION

Rehabilitation based on the International Classification of Functioning (ICF) can be described as an intervention/service/goal "to enable persons with health conditions experiencing or likely to experience disability to achieve and maintain optimal function."[13]

Initiation of CBR can be done by the top-down approach or bottom-up approach. In a top-down approach, an agency initiates the CBR outside of the community, and in a bottom-up approach, the activities are initiated, supported, and planned by the local community. Either way, community involvement is paramount for success. It is crucial that the community should be ready to accept, develop, and implement the program and the resources made available to do so.[14,15]

For a gainful CBR impact, it should be user-organized involving a local volunteer who understands local psychosocial and cultural scenario and has shown commitment. When clients are part of the decision-making process, it gives a sense of equality and empowerment too.

The CBR program has the following management steps[14]:

- Situational analysis
- Planning
- Implementation
- Evaluation

Situational Analysis

Before a CBR project initiates, ground analyses involving geographic, political, and demographic facts and figures are necessary to understand the local area. Stakeholders should be identified and involved early in the process of situational analysis, including local administrative offices and government scheme/service providers.

Random interviews with disabled persons and community leaders should be undertaken to motivate and promote their participation and also to assess the local priorities. Disabled People's Organization and civil society groups should be involved, to create a network and to find available resources. These groups can also help to advertise the cause, ensuring responses from government and other service provider agencies (advocacy).

The integrated, accessible health and health-related rehabilitation service delivery should have standardized protocols to refer clients to secondary and tertiary rehabilitation centers, along with the respective service coordinator.

Core CBR personnel/multipurpose rehabilitation worker's/CBR manager's role and job profile and responsibility should also be explained.

A meeting should be organized with all the stakeholders to identify a mutually agreed on priority to start the CBR work, and a possible appropriate solution is discussed for problems as they become evident.

Planning

During the early stages of planning of a rehabilitation program, it should be clear that the prioritized disability-related health issue that is addressed first will be the entry point. At this time, all the stakeholders should make certain of their free views, commitment, possible barriers, and solutions.

As Lord Kelvin quoted, "if you cannot measure it, you cannot improve it," therefore, short-term and long-term SMART goals made, that is, specific, measurable, attainable, relevant, and timely. Outcome indicators, measurable points, and outcomes of the program should be decided to evaluate in a specific timeframe and manner. Measurable goals and activities should be enumerated depending on the situational analysis.

After a specific objective analysis, a list of programmatic activities is generated. It also gives direction for resource analysis of the workforce, equipment, and supplies required. Three types of activities are prepared: rehabilitation activities directed toward the disabled and its family, supportive activities to facilitate rehabilitation and social support services, and development activities for capacity building. Activities should be relevant to the SMART goals established, for example, identification of clients, disability assessment, training family trainers, specific training like wheelchair transfers, and other related interventions. There is no preset draft to start an activity, start from the area of need, involve and expand, and invite the disabled and nondisabled community members to be part of the activity.

Three types of resources are looked for to meet the goal-oriented activity: human resource, material resource, and financial resource.

Human resource

Rehabilitation services should integrate with PHCs, because setting up an independent and parallel system will be a costly affair. The existing medical officer can take the role of supervising rehabilitation activities and referrals, and the cadre of multipurpose rehabilitation worker with the local volunteer (agent of change)[16] provides essential rehabilitation inputs for therapy, activities of daily living, and temporary orthotics using locally available materials.

People who are already in the primary health and social service model at the village level can be retrained and reassigned as multipurpose rehabilitation workers. The task shifting to alternative cadre in resource-poor areas is a promising option to deliver health-related rehabilitation services.[17,18] Development of such alternate cadres should be promoted, and outcomes should be researched for improvisation and learning. They will have to develop new skills over time as per local needs.[19,20]

Therapists, technicians, nurses, and health care assistants or community-based workers can also be trained as multipurpose workers with basic training in various aspects of rehabilitation services, like splint manufacturing or therapeutic exercises to provide rehabilitation services under supervision, while referring more complex and acute patients to more specialized rehabilitation centers at the district level or tertiary care centers.[21,22]

There is an inadequate supply of rehabilitation professionals in low- and middle-income countries,[23] even in developed regions like Australia and North America; there is a shortage of rehabilitation personnel in rural and remote areas.[24,25] In a resource-constrained area, staff skills rather than staff type should be considered to achieve the goal.

The other factor is that professionals who do not live in the community will stay for a short period only in the community and may not be able to dedicate adequate time to the community work. The multipurpose worker who comes from the community will commit for the long term. Professionals can come to advise, guide, and help in improving the skills of the local rehabilitation worker.[16]

There is ample evidence that multidisciplinary workforce professionals, like occupational therapists, physical therapists, rehabilitation technicians, speech and language therapists, social workers, psychologists, and physical medicine and rehabilitation specialists, can improve the rehabilitation outcome. Such a team can be made available at a referral center like secondary or tertiary rehabilitation health facilities, but a transdisciplinary/task-shifting approach is more practical for the grass root level in a low-resource area.[14]

A local village volunteer from the local community identified as "an agent of change" will help to facilitate rehabilitation interventions/services, raise advocacy and awareness, facilitate data collection, and guide the design of culturally appropriate measures. Most of the thriving community activities have been led and staffed by the local disabled persons. From their experience with the impairment and the local society, they know the problems, needs, and solutions.[16] The volunteer will do a home visit and work directly with the families and create a dynamic support system for the local disabled persons. An honorarium can be paid depending on the provision of funds.

Group activities and community interactions should be planned at a designated village area or neighborhood to promote social integration, small clusters of self-help, or parent groups, who can independently discuss and generate ideas or become family trainers to promote and execute rehabilitation training. The group can be supported and supervised by the midlevel multipurpose rehabilitation worker.

Material resources
Materials will include the type of facility, rehabilitation equipment, material, and space required for setting up the services. The premises of the primary health center can be used to reduce outlay, for better supervision and to integrate health/health-related rehabilitation services to the target community.

Aids and equipment should be adapted to the local culture and way of life, for example, the "Jaipur Foot," or below-knee prosthesis. The early below-knee prosthesis designed with the SACH foot was planned to fulfill western needs and was not able to suffice local needs/culture of Indian amputees. Prof. P.K. Sethi[26,27] innovated a new prosthesis often known as the "Jaipur Foot" in the 1970s, made of vulcanized rubber, leather, and aluminum sheet, all of which are quite commonly available at the village level. This prosthesis is adapted for the Indian culture of barefoot/floor activities and paddy field demands of agriculture workers and laborers; it remains the highest prescribed prosthesis in India.

Funds for such projects can come from local businesses, nongovernmental organizations, corporate houses, and various donors or agencies, for example, Bhagwan Mahaveer Viklang Sahayata Samiti, which mainly supports the "Jaipur Foot" project all over the world.

Financial resource

As Amartya Sen argued in "Poverty and famine: an essay on entitlement and deprivation" that "the supply chain is seldom affected by the paucity of funds but from inequalities built into mechanisms for distributing it, the bottleneck in the supply chain, asymmetric information, a mismatch in demand and supply."[28] Funds can always come for CBR activity, if the financial needs and sources can be restructured.

CBR is part of the primary health center for all administrative and financial matters.[12,28] Rehabilitation should not be considered as a population-specific intervention but an essential part of primary health care provisions under the Universal Health Coverage[29–31]; also, planning and priorities for rehabilitation involvement must conjugate with health data on disease and disability available in the health system. The multipurpose rehabilitation worker and the supervisor (primary health care physician of PHC) will propose the financial plan; the financial management should be transparent and accountable to implementing agencies, stakeholders, community, and civil society.

A detailed cost estimate must be done with the funding required at different phases, and stepwise funding, which is goal linked. The proposed draft should be reviewed by the financial department and agencies that will subsequently help to streamline the budget.

Sometimes self-finance aids and interventions are planned in the CBR, but in low-resource areas where poverty and social injustice are pervasive, it would not be fair to expect the poor to pay for it. Community contribution can not only be in the form of monetary contribution but also be a material donation or volunteering one's time for assistance to such projects.

Implementation

All necessary planned activities should be timed to produce the best results, so consultation with the local village volunteer or community member is done before finalizing. The village volunteer should act as a stimulant to the program rather than an end-of-line worker. They should be able to create a self-help group or parent groups as rehabilitation trainers who can later train the clients through their network.[16]

Collection of data and outcome reports/assessments and filing should be scheduled, and deadlines should be in place for proper monitoring. The source of verification for outcome assessments should also be defined beforehand. Detailed work plans should be communicated and discussed with the team and supervisors.

Recruitment/task shifting and the number of recruits will depend on the needs of the community. The multipurpose rehabilitation worker and the agent of change should be trained not only in rehabilitation-related health services but also in other aspects of rehabilitation as specified in the CBR matrix (see **Fig. 1**). The trainees should get input from all related professionals in a group setting, and it can end in accreditation or certificate. Staff development should be a continuing education activity for which various specialists, like physiatrists, physical therapists, occupational therapists, special education teacher, district rehabilitation officer, social worker, and rehabilitation technicians, can visit for few days at the local center based on their need.

Rehabilitation activity/networking can take place at someone's home, school, marketplace, village square, or health center.[16] Identification of clients, their disability, and service need should be identified along with primary health sensitization by the networking team.

Evaluation

It is the final cycle of management, and an ongoing process to determine outcomes, problem-solving, and restructuring/replanning. Timed evaluation gives us feedback on how much CBR-based multipronged process by integrating CBR with essential primary health care system was able to achieve, how efficiently the community intervention has worked, and what impact it has left in the short term and long term.

It will be carried out by the local team, including supervisor and results shared with governmental health/social agency, funding agency, and community leaders. A policy of transparency should be adopted in principles like providing greater disclosure, clarity, and accuracy in communication.

INTERNATIONAL CLASSIFICATION OF FUNCTIONING AND COMMUNITY-BASED REHABILITATION

ICF is an international framework and classification for functioning and disability, providing the technical infrastructure for recording, communicating, and measuring.[32,33] It can act as a framework to assess impairment, type of disability, needs, difficulties in activity and participation, environmental factors along with demographic and relative psychological factors. It can provide survey questions, a framework, and a checklist based on the needs of the program and can be used at all stages of the CBR management cycle.[34]

TELEREHABILITATION AND COMMUNITY-BASED REHABILITATION

Communication and related technologies like mobile, video conferencing, Internet, and gadgetry for telerehabilitation are powerful mechanisms that can add impetus to CBR services.[35,36] The team members can use it for communication, collective decision making, and sharing data. Mobile technology has become quite affordable, for example, owning a mobile phone with Internet services for a month may cost less than a dollar in India. If appropriate to the local community and service providers, it can be used for teleconsultations and guidance from rehabilitation professionals or multipurpose rehabilitation workers.[37,38] Moreover, for data collection and surveys, mobile operating system application-based protocols can be used,[39] like mICF (ICan Function Mobile Solution; icfmobile.org). Even though various studies have endorsed telerehabilitation efficacy and effectiveness, more research and funding are required to establish it as a reliable tool.[40,41]

SPECIALIZED REHABILITATION SERVICES AND REFERRALS

While providing specialized rehabilitation services, it is necessary that the provider or the health center have trained professionals or skilled community-based workers

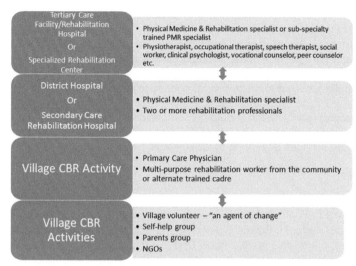

Fig. 2. PMR service structure and referral matrix. NGOs, nongovernmental organizations.

for competent services.[34] However, it would be too much to ask to have a multidisciplinary team at a district/provincial or community level in a resource-poor area, but when encountering a client with a unique or complex need, he or she should be referred to the next higher center for more focused and comprehensive management under a multidisciplinary team (**Fig. 2**). There is ample evidence that an inpatient program in a specialized service followed by outpatient services until rehabilitation goal achievement results in a better outcome and reduces mortality.[7]

There is also a worry that if community-rehabilitation service is not delivered by appropriately trained rehabilitation professionals that it may harm the health and functioning of people with disabilities in the long run. Therefore, it will be well advised that a CBR program should get planning, guidance, training, and management inputs from physical medicine and rehabilitation specialists to truly integrate CBR in the health system.[42]

CHALLENGES

Rehabilitation is a good investment and should be addressed solely through health services. Specific legislation and implementing rehabilitation-related services at the village/community level will not only need good governance but firm leadership. At the national level, low- and middle-income countries will have to take up a collaborative approach often termed "Health in All Policies" to create benefits across different sectors affecting health and beyond, not only to improve health and health-related rehabilitation but also to generate revenue to cover health/rehabilitation plans at the grass root level. Fiscal policies should be adopted to prevent and to cover treatment of illness, for example, compulsory health insurance for all building workers through builders to cover for illness/trauma, including rehabilitation interventions while promoting a safe workplace.[43,44]

Health priorities are always pushed toward acute health issues, and even insurance coverage has shifted more toward tertiary care rather than primary health and health-related rehabilitation,[43] which is quite visible when the facilities at corporate hospitals and village health centers are looked at. There is a dearth of knowledge among the policymakers about physical medicine and rehabilitation and related issues across all management levels.

To impart basic knowledge about disability, its management, and rehabilitation among health care professionals, including physicians, a primary module needs to be integrated into educational programs related to health care.[6] It will create sensitivity for the disability issues and make them proactive to intervene for or refer the disabled client.

Health-related rehabilitation should be compulsorily integrated with the health system, and collaboration should be created with vocational and social service providers to consolidate services according to CBR matrix.

REFERENCES

1. World Bank, World Health Organization. The world report on disability. Geneva (Switzerland): WHO Press; 2011.
2. Banks LM, Kuper H, Polack S. Poverty and disability in low- and middle-income countries: a systemic review. PLoS One 2017;12(12).
3. Mactaggert I, Kuper H, Murthy GVS, et al. Assessing health and rehabilitation needs of people with disabilities in Cameroon and India. Disabil Rehabil 2016; 38(18):1757–64.
4. WHO global disability action plan 2014-2021. Geneva (Switzerland): WHO Press; 2015.
5. Gutenbrunner C, Nugraha B. Principles of assessment of rehabilitation services in health systems: learning from experience. J Rehabil Med 2018;50:326–32.
6. Khan F, Owolabi MO, Amatysa B, et al. Challenges and barriers for implementation of the World Health Organization global disability action plan in low- and middle-income countries. J Rehabil Med 2018;50:367–76.
7. Furlan AD, Irvin E, Munhall C, et al. Rehabilitation service models for people with physical and/or mental disability in low- and middle-income countries: a systemic review. J Rehabil Med 2018;50:487–98.
8. Maya T. Reflections on community based rehabilitation. Psychol Developing Societies 2011;23(2):277–91.
9. Gutenbrunner C, Bickenbach J, Melvin J, et al. Strengthening health-related rehabilitation services at national level. J Rehabil Med 2018;50:317–25.
10. WHO, ILO, UNESCO, the International Disability and Development Consortium, IDDC. Community-based rehabilitation: CBR guidelines. Malta: Introductory Booklet. Geneva (Switzerland): WHO Press; 2010.
11. World Health Organization. People-centered and integrated health services: interim report. Geneva (Switzerland): WHO press; 2015.
12. Meyer T, Gutenbrunner C, Bickenbach J, et al. Towards a conceptual description of rehabilitation as a health strategy. J Rehabil Med 2011;43:765–9.
13. WHO global strategy on people-centered and integrated health services. Interim report. Geneva (Switzerland): WHO press; 2015.
14. WHO. International classification of functioning, disability and health. ICF, Geneva (Switzerland): World Health Organization; 2001.
15. Rehabilitation in health systems. Geneva (Switzerland): WHO press; 2017.
16. Community-Based Rehabilitation. CBR guidelines. Geneva (Switzerland): World Health Organization; 2010.
17. Werner D. Disabled village children. New Delhi: Voluntary Health Association of India; 1994.

18. Hasheem M, Boostrom C, MacLachlam M, et al. A systemic review of the effectiveness of alternative cadres in community based rehabilitation. Hum Resour Health 2012;10(20):1–8.
19. Chappel P, Johannameier C. The impact of community based rehabilitation as implemented by community rehabilitation facilitators on people with disabilities, their families and communities within South Africa. Disabil Rehabil 2009; 31(1):7–13.
20. Fulton BD, Scheffler RM, Sparkes SP, et al. Health workforce skill mix and task shifting in low income countries: a review of recent evidence. Hum Resour Health 2011;9:1.
21. Dubois CA, Singh D. From staff mix to skill mix and beyond: towards a systemic approach to health workforce management. Hum Resource Health 2009;1:1–9.
22. Stanmore E, Waterman H. Crossing professional and organizational boundaries: the implementation of generic rehabilitation assistants within three organizations in the northwest of England. Disabil Rehabil 2007;29:751–9.
23. Increasing access to health workers in remote and rural areas through improved retention: global policy recommendations. Geneva (Switzerland): WHO press; 2010.
24. Al Mahdy H. Rehabilitation and community services in Iran. Clinician Management 2002;11:57–60.
25. Wilson RD, Lewis SA, Murray PK. Trends in the rehabilitation therapist workforce in underserved areas: 1980–2000. J Rural Health 2009;25:26–32.
26. Sethi PK, Udawat MP, Kasliwal SC, et al. Vulcanized rubber foot for lower limb amputees. Prosthetics Orthotics Int 1978;2:125–36.
27. Sethi PK. The Knud Jensen Lecture. Technological choices in prosthetics and orthotics in developing countries. Prosthetics Orthotics Int 1989;13:117–24.
28. Poverty & famine: an essay on entitlement and deprivation. Oxford (England): Clarendon Press; 1981.
29. People-centered and integrated health services: an overview of the evidence: interim report. Geneva (Switzerland): WHO press; 2015.
30. Kamm CP, Schmid JP, Muri RM, et al. Interdisciplinary cardiovascular and neurologic outpatient rehabilitation in patients surviving transient ischemic attack or stroke with minor or no residual deficits. Arch Phys Med Rehabil 2014;95:656–62.
31. Emery EE, Lapidos S, Eisenstein AR, et al. The BRIGHTEN program: implementation and evaluation of a program to bridge resources of an interdisciplinary geriatric health team via electronic networking. Gerontologist 2012;52:857–65.
32. Jessep SA, Walsh NE, Ratcliffe J, et al. Long-term clinical benefits and costs of an integrated rehabilitation programme compared with outpatient physiotherapy for chronic knee pain. Physiotherapy 2009;95:94–102.
33. WHO. International classification on functioning, disability & health. Geneva (Switzerland): WHO; 2001.
34. Schneider M, Hartley S. International Classification of Functioning, Disability & Health (ICF) and CBR. In: Community-Based Rehabilitation (CBR) - a part of community development. University College London; 2006. p. 96–115.
35. Musoke G, Geiser P. Linking CBR, disability and rehabilitation. CBR Africa Network; 2013.
36. Seelman KD, Hartman LM. Telerehabilitation: policy issues and research tools. Int J Tele Rehabil 2009;1:47–58.
37. Taylor DM, Cameron JI, Walsh L, et al. Exploring the feasibility of video conference delivery of a self-management program to rural participants with stroke. Telemed E J Health 2009;15:646–54.

38. Fary F, Amatya B, Mannan H, et al. Neurorehabilitation in developing countries: a way forward. Phys Med Rehabil Int 2015;2:1070.
39. Lemaire ED, Boudrias Y, Greene G. Low-bandwidth, Internet-based videoconferencing for physical rehabilitation consultations. J Telemed Telecare 2001;7:82–9.
40. Sarfo FS, Adamu S, Awuah D, et al. Potential role of tele-rehabilitation to address barriers to implementation of physical therapy among West African stroke survivors: a cross-sectional survey. J Neurol Scie 2017;381:203–8.
41. Kairy D, Lehoux P, Vincent C, et al. A systematic review of clinical outcomes, clinical process, healthcare utilization and costs associated with telerehabilitation. Disabil Rehabil 2009;31:427–47.
42. Meyer T, Gutenbrunner C, Kiekens C, et al. ISPRM discussion paper: proposing a conceptual description of health-related rehabilitation services. J Rehabil Med 2014;46:1–6.
43. Seijas VA, Lugo LH, Cano B, et al. Understanding community-based rehabilitation and the role of physical and rehabilitation medicine. Eur J Phys Rehabil Med 2018;54(1):90–9.
44. Jamison DT, Gelband H, Horton S, et al. Disease control priorities, third edition. Washington, DC: World Bank; 2017.

Appropriate Assistive Technology for Developing Countries

María Luisa Toro-Hernández, PhD[a],*, Padmaja Kankipati, PhD[b],
Mary Goldberg, PhD[c], Silvana Contepomi, PT[d],
Denise Rodrigues Tsukimoto, OT[e], Nathan Bray, PhD[f]

KEYWORDS

- Assistive technology • Access • Evidence-based • Human rights • Policy
- Service provision • Workforce

KEY POINTS

- For many people with decreased functioning, assistive technology is required to participate as independently as possible in the activities that one values.
- It is a human right to provide proximate access to appropriate assistive technology service provision for those who need it.
- Coordinated efforts to advance policy, provision, products, and personnel based on up-to-date and reliable understanding of the population's needs are urgent in the developing world.
- Deep understanding of the nuances and particularities of each context are a prerequisite to progress.
- International cooperation and technical assistance are needed to reach the most vulnerable as quickly as possible.

INTRODUCTION

The International Classification of Functioning, Disability, and Health defines the spectrum between functioning and disability as the result of a complex interaction between

Disclosure Statement: The authors have nothing to disclose.
[a] School of Physiotherapy, Universidad CES, Calle 10A #22-04, Medellín, Colombia;
[b] Specialized Mobility Operations & Innovation, 804, Brigade Rubix, No. 20, HMT Main Road, Yeshwanthpura, Bangalore 560022, India; [c] International Society of Wheelchair Professionals, Department of Rehabilitation Science and Technology, Human Engineering Research Laboratories, University of Pittsburgh, 6425 Penn Avenue Suite 400, Pittsburgh, PA 15206, USA;
[d] Asociación Argentina de Tecnología Asistiva (AATA), Francia 3166, San Isidro 1642, Argentina;
[e] Physical Medicine and Rehabilitation Institute (IMREA), Hospital das Clinicas, University of Sao Paulo, IMREA Rua Diderot, 43, Sao Paulo, Sao Paulo CEP: 04116030, Brazil; [f] School of Health Sciences, Bangor University, Bangor, Gwynedd LL57 2EF, UK
* Corresponding author.
E-mail address: mhtoro@ces.edu.co

Phys Med Rehabil Clin N Am 30 (2019) 847–865
https://doi.org/10.1016/j.pmr.2019.07.008

an individual with a health condition and his or her context that may result in activity limitations and participation restrictions.[1] The rapid rise in the aging population and the increased prevalence of noncommunicable diseases translates to a rise in the number of individuals living with long-term impaired functioning.[1,2] Assistive technology (AT) is an umbrella term that describes products and services that enhance individuals' functioning and participation; including systems, services, products, devices, equipment, and software.[1,3,4] Therefore, AT promotes independence both in people with disabilities across their life span[5] and in older adults.[6] Eighty percent of people with disabilities live in the developing world[7] and the World Health Organization (WHO) estimates that approximately 1 in 10 individuals who need AT, have access to it.[8] Women, children, individuals with multiple impairments (eg, people who are deafblind[9]), and people in emergency and disaster situations are at higher risk of exclusion.[10–12] The adoption of the United Nations Convention on the Rights of Persons with Disabilities (CRPD) in 2006 recognizes access to appropriate and affordable AT as a human right,[13] resulting in increased awareness and advocacy worldwide.[5,14,15] The CRPD has been ratified by 175 United Nations Member States, who are thus obligated to ensure affordable AT is available to all individuals in need.[8] Governments therefore have an obligation to coordinate high-volume AT procurement and import tax waivers to reduce costs, subsequently improving AT coverage. Nevertheless, persistent challenges remain to the fulfillment of commitment to the aging and disability community ensuring equitable access to appropriate AT.[8] The Sustainable Development Goals call for inclusive actions to leave no one behind and to design poverty alleviation and development programs inclusive to people with disabilities and older adults.[15–17] Hence, AT can be described both as a mediator and moderator of sustainable development.[15,17]

Access is a complex concept that involves availability, physical accessibility, adequate supply, affordability, and acceptability.[18] Although AT products are essential, as illustrated in **Fig. 1**, successful access depends on integrated efforts related to end users (the "people"), provision, personnel, products, and policy, deemed the 5 Ps by the World Health Organization's Global Cooperation on Assistive Technology (WHO GATE).[19,20] These 5Ps are unique to each context.[21]

This article briefly details (1) AT types and progress toward making them globally available; (2) AT challenges in developing countries, including cost-effectiveness of AT; (3) select country snapshots demonstrating AT systems in practice; and (4) opportunities in improving access to appropriate AT and service provision.

TYPES OF ASSISTIVE TECHNOLOGY

To assist governments, the WHO published the Assistive Priority List (APL) that includes 50 products, developed via a global Delphi study, across a variety of AT types.[6] Governments are urged to adapt and adopt the APL according to their national needs (people).[6] However this may be overwhelming for governments; the ISO AT classification system (**Table 1**) could be a useful guide.

In the absence of adequate access to appropriate AT, do-it-yourself (DIY) initiatives are becoming more popular, with the democratization of information and tools (eg, 3-dimensional printing). The risk of DIY AT is the possibility of inappropriate products reaching end users.[22]

CHALLENGES IN ASSISTIVE TECHNOLOGY IN DEVELOPING COUNTRIES

Challenges including limited policy governing supply and provision, an insufficient workforce, limited training capacity, and limited product supply and enforced

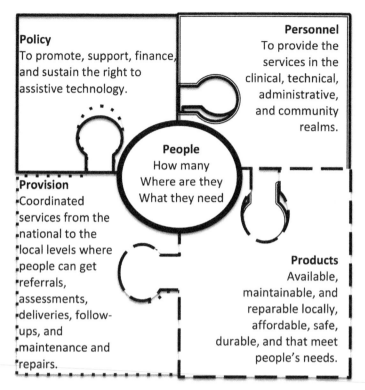

Fig. 1. The 5Ps required for appropriate access to AT. (*Adapted from* World Health Organization. Global Cooperation on Assistive Technology - About us. July 2018. Available at: http://www.who.int/phi/implementation/assistive_technology/phi_gate/en/. Accessed September 4, 2018; with permission.)

standards accumulate to create a difficult environment to ensure appropriate AT is provided to users, especially in developing countries.[23–26]

International human rights legislation can provide a helpful framework, but national examples of legislation and policy governing AT are limited. For example, South Africa Guidelines for AT Service Standardization,[27] Chile "Funding orientations for AT" 2018,[28] and Nordic Countries Provision of AT 2007[29] provide an upper-middle income, and high-income examples, respectively, of national level guidelines. Papua New Guinea offers Draft Guidelines from 2016[30] as a lower middle income example. The global landscape is not as promising. Without mandated policies through national legislation, providers are unlikely to pursue and maintain certification, and if governments do finance AT, they are unlikely to be aware of or adhere to product standards.

Without governing policy, training is unlikely to be required for AT providers. Inadequate training of rehabilitation or community health care providers, who are often the first point of people contact,[31] can result in inappropriate provision, which has negative impacts on quality of life, health, safety, and other human rights.[32–36] Trained service providers (personnel) have the potential to reduce AT users' prevalence of secondary health conditions and may contribute to reducing disparities.[32] *Building capacity goes hand in hand with the integration of these services into existing health care programs for ensuring equitable access to appropriate AT.*[37,38]

Table 1
Assistive technology products classification according to ISO 9999:2016

ISO 9999:2016 Product Class	Product Examples (Not Comprehensive but Intended to Illustrate the Vast Range, One Product May Belong to More than One Class)
For measuring, supporting, training or replacing body functions	Pressure relief wheelchair cushion (for tissue integrity)
For education and for training in skills	Mobile application to train in everyday activities Paint brush with thick handle to train in painting skills
Attached to the body for supporting neuromusculoskeletal or movement related functions and replacing anatomic structures	Below-knee prosthesis Spine orthosis
For self-care activities and participation in self-care	Kid's protective cap One-handed buttoning devices and fasteners
For activities and participation relating to personal mobility and transportation	Van that can be driven from a power wheelchair Elbow crutches White cane
For domestic activities and participation in domestic life	Easy-grip garden fork Fixed food cutting board
Furnishings, fixtures, and other assistive products for supporting activities in indoor and outdoor human-made environments	Chair with special mechanism to assist the person to stand Kid's floor seats
For communication and information management	Magnifier lens Face-to-face communication software Computer joystick
For controlling, carrying, moving, and handling objects and devices	Reacher Small table on wheels
For controlling, adapting, or measuring elements of physical environments	Noise reduction board Barometer
For work activities and participation in employment	Workplace mat for reducing vibration Height-adjustable work bench
For recreation and leisure	Switch-activated toys Blind-soccer ball

Data from EASTIN. Guided search – assistive products. Available at: http://www.eastin.eu/en/searches/products/iso.

In addition to policy, training, and workforce concerns, products also may be limited, and those that are available may not meet standards.[19] Two key barriers to ensuring universal AT provision are cost and availability: the low production levels of AT within many developing countries leads to increased scarcity, subsequently the specialized nature of AT interventions leads to small markets and, thus, higher costs.[39] Few countries govern product supply; simply making the technology available to a population is insufficient, as inappropriate products can still be delivered to the user.[19]

It is evident that the relative cost-effectiveness of most AT in developing nations is unclear, predominantly due to an almost nonexistent evidence base. To understand the efficiency of different AT equipment and services, it is important to not only understand their cost but also the subsequent benefits they provide for AT users. By exploring how best to measure the cost and benefits of AT, health economists can help to determine which technologies and devices offer the most cost-effective method of improving the quality of life and health of people with impairments. Furthermore, by assessing a range of comparable AT, incremental costs and benefits of competing alternatives can be examined. Thus, decisions about provision can be guided by incremental cost-effectiveness evidence. In developing countries, it is imperative that ATs are low cost, durable, and simple to produce/repair locally. However, the relationship between cost and user outcomes is equally important, as the relative value for money of AT can be determined only by examining the cost per unit of effect. Furthermore, the perspective of such analysis needs to be explicit, as cost-effectiveness estimates are likely to vary depending on whether a government, charity, or individual is expected to pay for their own AT. Methods of economic evaluation need to be imbedded in future research in this context, and seen as an integral part of the evaluation of AT interventions and services across the world.

To examine the relationship between costs and outcomes, health economists commonly undertake economic evaluations. Health economics and the economic evaluation of health technologies is becoming increasingly influential in the financing and analysis of health care across the world. One of the predominant approaches to economic evaluation is cost-effectiveness analysis (CEA), which compares alternative methods of achieving a predetermined outcome; for example, additional life years. CEA directly examines the relationship between costs and effects (ie, benefits) for a specified intervention and comparator.[40] The intervention that incurs the least cost and highest benefit (or equal benefit) is determined the most cost-effective intervention.[41] An incremental cost-effectiveness ratio may be calculated to compare relative costs and incremental benefits of differing but comparative interventions. CEA relies on a single outcome measure, as cost cannot be attributed to 2 separate outcomes or when outcomes are mutually exclusive (ie, extended life but decreased quality of life).[41] Direct comparison between the value of costs and effects is not possible.[40,42]

To date, the application of methods of economic evaluation to AT has been limited, particularly in low and middle income countries. This is partially because of the difficulties of applying traditional methods of economic evaluation in the context of AT provision, where outcomes are often less explicitly defined compared with pharmaceutical and surgical interventions. Although AT costs are frequently reported in this context,[43] specific cost-effectiveness analyses are few and far between. The evidence available in the developing world on AT is mostly focused on mobility and vision devices and more than half of the studies are observational designs.[44]

The way the various challenges manifest in practice is context-dependent as revealed in the following country snapshots.

COUNTRY SNAPSHOTS

As mentioned previously, AT products are essential but not sufficient to guarantee the right to appropriate AT.[19,20] The brief country snapshots help the reader grasp the complexities, challenges, and opportunities that are entangled in each of the contexts. These snapshots are not representative of the developing world as a whole, as each context is unique.

Argentina: Community Empowerment to Provide Assistive Technology to the Most Vulnerable

Argentina is an emerging economy, similar to most of the countries in the region and shares corruption scandals that make poverty and violence evident. Currently,

27.3% of Argentina's population lives in poverty,[45] and disability is prevalent in 10.2% of the population.[46] Since 2001, the Ministry of Health has managed the unified national disability registry, which provides the disability certificate that includes the cause of disability, level, and rehabilitation services.[47] This law allows for the provision of AT products, but most remote and poor places lack appropriate processes to guarantee the rights of people with disabilities.

An example of a vulnerable group in Argentina is the indigenous group Wichi that lives in the region Banda Sur del Chaco Salteño. This region accounts for a higher rate of childhood malnourishment and poverty than the national average.[48] A health community strengthening program led by social workers identified several cases of children with mobility impairments laying on the floor all day because of lack of appropriate AT. To promote the rights of these children, by providing access to appropriate AT,[13] a pilot project based on the WHO Community-Based Rehabilitation[49] (CBR) and the 8-steps-Wheelchair provision[33] started in 2016. Two social workers and 1 physical therapist (trained in the WHO Wheelchair Service Provision Packages[50]) designed and carried out the pilot program (**Fig. 2**).

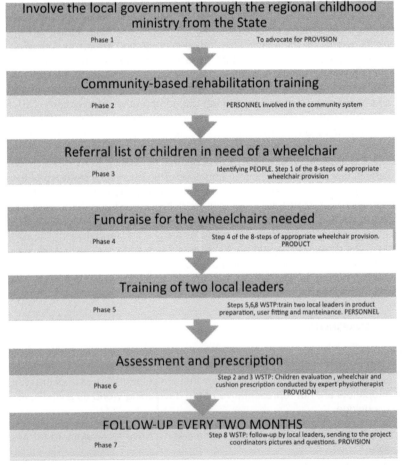

Fig. 2. Pilot CBR project to improve AT access considering people, personnel, provision, and products in the Wichi community, Argentina.

LESSONS LEARNED

- 21 children have received an appropriate wheelchair and training on its use and on postural care (**Fig. 3**).
- An increase in the number of cases of children requiring wheelchairs may indicate families having children at home without any community involvement.
- Fulfillment of the initial project goal, that is, access to appropriate AT, led to increased community participation that resulted in new needs becoming evident (eg, ramps, alternative communication solutions, toy adaptation). Although the CBR project focused on the AT element of the health component, it contributed to building awareness about promotion of inclusive development strategies in this community.

Steps forward: The program will train several health agents who have been helping with users' assessment and product prescription. The government has started to offer more training opportunities in CBR that promote inclusion.

Brazil: Public Health Commitment to Foster Progress in Rehabilitation

The 2000 Demographic Census reported that 14.5% of the Brazilian population had a disability, which rose to 23.9% in 2010. There is an increased demand for rehabilitation services and technologies.[51] Strengthening the provision of rehabilitation services and ensuring their proper funding is critical to guarantee that rehabilitation is available and affordable to those who need it.[52] Public health in Brazil has 2 distinct phases, and the creation of the Unified Health System (SUS for its name in Portuguese) is the watershed of these phases. Before the creation of the SUS in 1988, health was restricted to a portion of the population that had social insurance. Public health actions were of a preventive and community nature, with few health care exceptions focused on specific diseases or population groups, and assistance to people with disabilities was performed by philanthropic institutions.[53,54] In the 1988 Constitution, health was recognized as every citizen's right that must be guaranteed by the government.[53,54] Efforts have been made to increase the quality, equity, and economic accessibility of services.[52] The financing of SUS by the federal, state, and municipal governments should promote the collection and transfer of necessary resources in order to guarantee the universality and completeness of the system. Underfunding of SUS results in difficulties in meeting population demands and providing quality services to the population.

Even in the face of these difficulties, through the commitment of professionals and managers in the area of public health and the participation of various

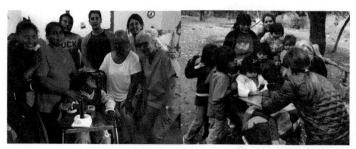

Fig. 3. Left, Ser and his mother, community workers, and expert rehabilitation mentor professionals. Right, team leader and user exploring an augmentative communication App. (*Courtesy of* Silvana Contepomi, PT, San Isidro, Argentina.)

stakeholders; exemplary actions and quality services have been developed, albeit with greater concentration in the urban central areas, including the following:

- Development of national guidelines for the care of people with disabilities based on scientific evidence to guide rehabilitation actions.
- Evaluation and delivery of quality orthoses, prostheses, and mobility aids through the SUS in rehabilitation reference centers.
- Development of research projects and introduction of new technologies through academic studies and research/innovation promotion agencies.
- The formation of a state level rehabilitation network in São Paulo, to provide health care coverage and educational and research actions; including a Mobile Rehabilitation Unit.

Rehabilitation research and development efforts within the public health system, have resulted in the following: (1) robotic technology for functional improvement of the limbs; (2) application of virtual reality and biofeedback by surface electromyography; (3) evaluations and therapies with neuromodulation; and (4) application of functional electrical stimulation, shock waves, and other physical treatment agents. Numerous government-assisted efforts conducted have resulted in the development and use of digital accessibility and augmentative communication resources; vocational courses, therapeutic workshops, and inclusion activities; and a Paralympic Center, to name a few. Continuing education initiatives for rehabilitation professionals ensure they remain up-to-date with new developments resulting in improved services.

Steps forward: Two types of actions are needed for successful implementation of rehabilitation technology.

- People with disabilities, caregivers, and undergraduate and postgraduate students, and the community as a whole need to be trained on appropriate AT usage (**Fig. 4**).
- All stakeholders (eg, end users, government ministries, social institutions, industry) need to coordinate for effective implementation.

Colombia: Significant Policy Advances, Need for Greater Coordination and Implementation

Colombia has a population of 45.5 million,[55] is an upper-middle income economy, and has one of the largest inequalities in the region: 26.9% of its population lives below the

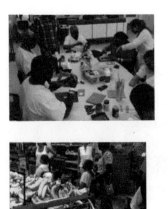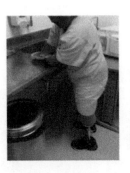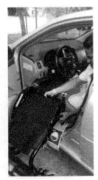

Fig. 4. AT users receiving training at a rehabilitation center in Brazil. (*Courtesy of* Physical Medicine and Rehabilitation Institute, Sao Paulo, Brazil.)

poverty line.[56] Its more than 60 years of internal conflict has resulted in more than 7.9 million people internally displaced and more than 11,000 landmine victims.[57,58] Preliminary data from the 2018 population census report that 7.2% live with a disability.[55]

The legal framework in Colombia has a rights-based approach, it has a young constitution (1991) that prohibits discrimination based on race, gender, ethnicity, religion, and disability and mandates the government to protect these vulnerable groups.[59] A peculiarity of the context is that for a law to be enforced, after enacted by the congress, it must be ruled by the executive branch, posing significant bureaucratic barriers toward the implementation of new enacted laws. The country has made significant strides toward universal health coverage (UHC), 94.36% of the country's population is covered by a mandatory health care plan,[60] but effective access to services remains a challenge and constantly requires legal appeal.[61] There are several policies and programs from before the CRPD that have impacted access to AT:

- Since 2001 the Relay Center provides, at no cost, online video-to-voice relay calls, online Colombian Sign Language (CSL) interpretation, and promotes CSL.[62]
- The National Disability System (2007), coordinated by the Interior Ministry, was created to articulate work between the public sector and civil society organizations to advocate and inform public policy and its implementation at the municipal, departmental, and national levels.[63]
- Since 2007, the mandatory health care plan has provided access to hearing aids, external lenses (out-of-pocket charges for the frame, filters, and protections), and prosthetics and orthotics,[64] including assessment and fitting services. Wheelchairs, cushions, and therapeutic footwear were explicitly excluded from the plan.[64]

The country signed (2009) and ratified (2011) the CRPD, which was later enacted in the Disability law (2013) and a National Disability Public Policy.[65] After the ratification of the CRPD, the following changes were made:

- The Ministry of Health (MoH) shall define, validate, implement, and evaluate the national comprehensive rehabilitation model.[66] This has the potential of creating an umbrella strategy that coordinates all the advances in AT.
- The National CBR guidelines, published in 2014, promote coordination between the MoH and community agents (including people with disabilities) to facilitate access and maintenance of AT.[67] Little is known about the implementation.[68]
- The Ministry of Information and Telecommunications acquired a national license (2013), for the screen-reader JAWS and the screen magnifier MAGIC, allowing more than 570,000 free downloads across the country by December 2017.[69,70]
- Highlights of a new health care law (2015) aimed to improve equitable access to health[71,72]:
  ○ Prosthetic and orthotic products and personnel need to comply with regulatory standards and licensing.[73,74]
  ○ Although speech therapy is covered, there is no mention of Augmentative and Alternative Communication services and devices.[71]
  ○ The MoH is mandated to provide funding to support AT Banks (ATB) designed to provide products that are excluded from the mandatory health plan to the poorest citizens (few being operational).[73]
  ○ MoH indicated that Braille boards should be provided by the Ministry of Education and incontinence pads by municipal or provincial local authorities, without specifying which entity.[75]

- In 2015, the Military forces enacted AT guidelines, including requirements on personnel, provision, and products.[76]
- Since 2016, the National Television Authority mandates the implementation of closed caption in national, provincial, and local public television.[77]
- In 2017, the Ministry of Education (MoE) enacted the decree for students with disabilities to have an individual reasonable accommodation plan (inclusive of AT), with the national government providing funds[78] and the local education authorities responsible for implementation.[78,79]
- The National Institute for the Blind (MoE) launched the free virtual library for people with visual impairment, allowing access to audio books and accessible digital content via mobile and Web browsing.[80]
- The Ministry of Labor passed the public employment decree (2017) that mandates local, provincial, and national governments to reserve a quota for employees with disability. Each public entity would be in charge of the needed reasonable accommodations.[81]

Fig. 5 synthesizes the national policy advances made and the challenges toward local implementation. Poor policy implementation is evident, as people with disabilities still face disproportionate low education, employment, and health outcomes.[82] Public implementation efforts still fail to reach the most vulnerable, international nongovernmental organizations (NGOs) (eg, International Committee of the Red Cross, Humanity for Inclusion, and World Vision) still play a role in providing access to prosthetics, orthotics, and wheelchairs to conflict survivors and people in rural communities.[83–85] The civil society shadow report to the United Nations states there is a lack of sufficient trained personnel related to rehabilitation, no care pathways, and those in rural areas have no access to professionals and services they need.[86,87]

Steps forward: The National Disability System poses a great opportunity to coordinate and unite the currently fragmented policy, infrastructure, and services with the goal of ensuring a widespread availability of appropriate AT as close as possible to their living location. It is urgent to conduct coordinated and financed

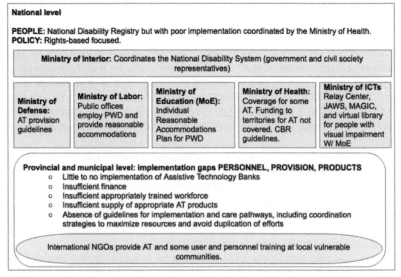

Fig. 5. Colombian AT-related national policy framework and territorial implementation gaps. PWD, people with disabilities.

capacity-building efforts on the personnel, provision, and product aspects to implement the legal framework advances. This could be designed with technical assistance from national experts (eg, Ministries of Defense) and the WHO[88] to achieve the CRPD mandate with regard to AT.

INDIA: INTERNATIONAL COOPERATION AND COLLABORATION SUPPORTING SUSTAINABLE INNOVATION

The Disabilities Act (2016) is the most recent comprehensive law in terms of nondiscrimination against persons with disabilities and obligates the corporate sector to ensure equal employment opportunity is provided. *However, little has been mentioned in terms of access to AT apart from the onus of provision lies as an obligation of the private employer.* The perception of disability in India has long been held as a social welfare concern. The Disability Act (2016) is indicative of the changing paradigm from a charitable model to that of a human rights issue.

One of the largest government financial aid programs for procuring AT is through the Assistance to Disabled Persons for Purchasing/Fitting of aids/Appliances (ADIP) scheme. The largest agency implementing the ADIP scheme is the Artificial Limbs Manufacturing Corporation of India (ALIMCO), a public sector undertaking. ALIMCO provides a range of AT products (eg, crutches, wheelchair, walking cane, braille slate, hearing aids). Products are provided through various fitting centers and donations through camps run in the rural and semi-urban areas of India, thereby establishing it as the largest national distributor of AT. Recent developments include new products and capacity-building efforts for ALIMCO staff, which will positively impact product and service quality.[89] **Fig. 6** illustrates this technology transfer scheme.

An example that showcases a successful collaborative effort of a sustainable innovation is the ReMotion Knee, which retails at approximately 80 USD. Now led by D-Rev, a nonprofit company, ReMotion Knee is currently being fitted in the Jaipur

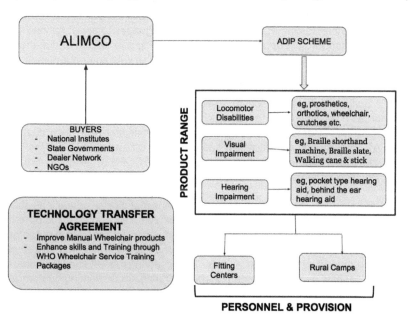

Fig. 6. AT transfer scheme between India's public agency for AT provision and an international NGO.

foot clinic and the company is currently establishing partnerships with prosthetics providers globally, expanding access to people with disabilities in India and beyond.[90]

Steps forward: Although the recent legislation is a step in the right direction to be more compliant with the CRPD, national standards for products and services need to be adopted according to global standards to ensure quality of services and products improve. In addition, successful implementation of policies requires a collective approach from all stakeholders.

OPPORTUNITIES IN THE ROAD AHEAD

As evidenced in the snapshots, countries are pursuing and experiencing unique pathways in ensuring appropriate AT products and service provisions for all. To address any of the challenges presented, awareness-raising strategies must be implemented: the benefits of AT and appropriate service provision should be known by different stakeholders that work with people with activity limitations across their life span: people with disabilities and their organizations, older adults, rehabilitation professionals, gerontologists, psychologists, educators, health agents, community health care workers, engineers, and designers. In addition to WHO open-source resources, there are other freely available knowledge and product platforms that are in several languages (*EASTIN*), Spanish (*CEAPAT, CIAPAT*), and English (*AbleNET*).

Next, political will and a high level of engagement are necessary. Tajikistan, with the polio outbreak in 2010, was able to establish a national rehabilitation framework, including AT, in less than 10 years.[88] In addition to the high-level commitment, they were able to succeed with technical assistance from WHO and international development funds from the United States.[88] WHO GATE has invested in identifying tools and helpful case studies related to AT policy,[20] and the International Society of Wheelchair Professionals (ISWP) has developed a policy toolkit for stakeholders who are influencing national policy decisions related to wheelchairs.[91]

Related to personnel capacity building, WHO has published a series of open-source Wheelchair Service Training Packages in multiple languages to assist nations in fulfilling the CRPD mandate of supporting providers' training and help to bridge the gap in training disparity across developing countries.[33,50] In developing countries, standard in-person training may be inaccessible, but in some cases, online learning has addressed various challenges of in-person training, such as limited access and high cost.[92,93] Building from this success, WHO GATE is developing a series of online, open-source AT modules that focus on AT represented in the WHO Priority Assistive Technologies list.[94] Complementary assessments, certification, and accreditation that validate AT competency and capacity, such as those offered by ISWP,[95] the International Society for Prosthetics and Orthotics,[96] and CECOPS (Community Equipment Code of Practice Scheme)[97] may institute quality control throughout the rehabilitation system.

Related to products, market shaping (interventions that aim to reduce long-term demand and supply imbalances and reach a sustainable equilibrium) has the potential to address breakdowns in the health care market and support better health outcomes for people in developing countries.[98] The US Agency for International Development (USAID) recommends 5 simple steps, including observing market shortcomings, diagnosing root causes, assessing market-shaping options, implementing customized interventions, and measuring results.[99] USAID's ATScale: A Global Partnership for Assistive Technology project, has taken a deeper dive into rehabilitation technology specifically, and aims to help 500 million people get the AT they need by 2030 through service delivery and market-shaping approaches; creating partnerships with the private sector to build and serve markets in the lowest-resource countries; supporting the development of country plans for greater access; and catalyzing innovation to design and introduce suitable AT where needed.[100] In developing countries, such as Brazil, where local production of AT has been established, the use of readily available indigenous resources facilitates low-cost AT solutions, as excessive import costs can be avoided as well as abandonment due to lack of repair components.[43] Furthermore, the mass production of AT in countries such as India has led to lower production costs and increased opportunities for international exports.[43] Governments also should remove or reduce import taxes on relevant materials and AT to ensure that population need for AT does not outstrip availability.

Last, robust research, monitoring, and evaluation plans must be created and followed to be able to build and strengthen the evidence that is lacking and that the global AT sector needs.[19]

REFERENCES

1. World Health Organization. International classification of functioning, disability and health: ICF. Geneva (Switzerland): World Health Organization; 2001.
2. World Health Organization. World report on ageing and health. Geneva (Switzerland): World Health Organization; 2015.
3. [PDF] ISO 9999:2016. Available at: https://www.sis.se/api/document/preview/920988/.
4. World Health Organization. Global cooperation on assistive technology. World Health Organization. Available at: http://www.who.int/phi/implementation/assistive_technology/phi_gate/en/. Accessed August 16, 2018.
5. Borg J, Berman-Bieler R, Khasnabis C, et al. Assistive technology for children with disabilities: creating opportunities for education, inclusion and participation. Geneva (Switzerland): World Health Organization and UNICEF; 2015. Available at: https://www.unicef.org/disabilities/files/Assistive-Tech-Web.pdf.
6. World Health Organization. Priority assistive products list. Geneva (Switzerland): World Health Organization; 2016.
7. World Health Organization. World report on disability. Geneva (Switzerland): World Health Organization; 2011.
8. WHO | Seventy-first World Health Assembly adopts resolution on assistive technology. Available at: http://www.who.int/phi/implementation/assistive_technology/71stWHA-adopts-resolution-on-assistive-technology/en/. Accessed August 30, 2018.
9. World Federation of the Deafblind. At risk of exclusion from CRPD and SDGs implementation: inequality and persons with deafblindness. Oslo (Norway): World Federation of the Deafblind; 2018. Available at: http://www.internationaldisabilityalliance.org/sites/default/files/wfdb_complete_initial_global_report_september_2018.pdf. Accessed September 10, 2019.
10. Disability-inclusive Humanitarian Action | United Nations Enable. United Nations - Disability. Available at: https://www.un.org/development/desa/disabilities/issues/whs.html. Accessed October 24, 2018.
11. UNICEF. The state of the world's children 2013: children with disabilities. New York: UNICEF; 2013. Available at: https://www.unicef.org/sowc2013/files/SWCR2013_ENG_Lo_res_24_Apr_2013.pdf.
12. United Nations. Report of the special rapporteur on the rights of persons with disabilities. New York: United Nations; 2018. Available at: https://www.ohchr.org/Documents/Issues/Disability/A_73_161_EN.pdf.

13. United Nations. Convention on the rights of persons with disabilities. 2006. Available at: http://www.un.org/disabilities/documents/convention/convoptprot-e.pdf.

14. Borg J, Larsson S, Östergren P. The right to assistive technology: for whom, for what, and by whom? Disabil Soc 2011;26(2):151–67.

15. Tebbutt E, Brodmann R, Borg J, et al. Assistive products and the Sustainable Development Goals (SDGs). Global Health 2016;12(1):79.

16. Morgon Banks L, Polack S. The economic costs of exclusion and gains of inclusion of people with disabilities: evidence from low and middle income countries. International Centre for Evidence in Disability, cbm, and London School of Hygiene & Tropical Medicine. Available at: https://www.iapb.org/wp-content/uploads/CBM_Costs-of-Exclusion-and-Gains-of-Inclusion-Report_2015.pdf. Accessed September 10, 2019.

17. United Nations. Sustainable Development Goals. 2017. Available at: https://www.un.org/sustainabledevelopment/sustainable-development-goals/. Accessed September 10, 2019.

18. Gulliford M, Figueroa-Munoz J, Morgan M, et al. What does "access to health care" mean? J Health Serv Res Policy 2002;7(3):186–8.

19. Smith RO, Scherer MJ, Cooper R, et al. Assistive technology products: a position paper from the first global research, innovation, and education on assistive technology (GREAT) summit. Disabil Rehabil Assist Technol 2018;13(5):473–85.

20. WHO | global cooperation on assistive technology - about us. Available at: http://www.who.int/phi/implementation/assistive_technology/phi_gate/en/. Accessed September 4, 2018.

21. Global research, innovation and education in assistive technology. Geneva (Switzerland): World Health Organization; 2017. Available at: http://apps.who.int/iris/bitstream/handle/10665/259746/WHO-EMP-IAU-2017.16-eng.pdf;jsessionid=385451B25A6EA35BDDC725847B45A1DA?sequence=1.

22. Grott R. Will 3D printers make our profession obsolete? Arlington: Rehabilitation Engineering & Assistive Technology Society of North America; 2015. Available at: https://www.resna.org/blog/will-3d-printers-make-our-profession-obsolete. Accessed November 20, 2018.

23. Economic Commission for Latin America and the Caribbean. Social panorama of Latin America 2012 - Cepal. Santiago (Chile): United Nations. Available at: https://www.cepal.org/en/publications/1248-social-panorama-latin-america-2012. Accessed September 10, 2019.

24. McSweeney E, Gowran RJ. Wheelchair service provision education and training in low and lower middle income countries: a scoping review. Disabil Rehabil Assist Technol 2019;14(1):33–45.

25. Who WB. World report on disability. Geneva (Switzerland): WHO; 2011.

26. Banks LM, Kuper H, Polack S. Poverty and disability in low- and middle-income countries: a systematic review. PLoS One 2017;12(12):e0189996.

27. Standardisation of provision of assistive devices in South Africa: a guideline for use in the public sector. Available at: http://uhambofoundation.org.za/new_wp/wp-content/uploads/2016/06/standardisation_of_provision_of_assistive_devices_in_south_.pdf. Accessed September 10, 2019.

28. Ministerio de Desarrollo Social y Familia. Tecnologias para la inclusion. Available at: https://www.senadis.gob.cl/pag/461/1649/proceso_de_financiamiento_ayudas_tecnicas_2018. Accessed September 10, 2019.

29. Nordic Cooperation on Disability Issues. 2007. Provision of assistive technology in the Nordic countries, second edition. Available at: http://sid.usal.es/idocs/F8/FDO20694/provisionassistivetechnology.pdf. Accessed September 10, 2019.

30. National guidelines on the provision of assistive technology in Papua New Guinea. Available at: http://pak.wheelchairnetwork.org/wp-content/uploads/2018/07/Papau-New-Guinea-Draft-2016.pdf. Accessed September 10, 2019.

31. Vasan A, Mabey DC, Chaudhri S, et al. Support and performance improvement for primary health care workers in low- and middle-income countries: a scoping review of intervention design and methods. Health Policy Plan 2017;32(3):437–52.

32. Visagie S, Scheffler E, Schneider M. Policy implementation in wheelchair service delivery in a rural South African setting. Afr J Disabil 2013;2(1):63.

33. World Health Organization, WHO. Guidelines on the provision of manual wheelchairs in less resourced settings. World Health Organization; 2008.

34. Universal declaration of human rights. Available at: http://www.un.org/en/universal-declaration-human-rights/. Accessed August 29, 2018.

35. Toro ML, Eke C, Pearlman J. The impact of the World Health Organization 8-steps in wheelchair service provision in wheelchair users in a less resourced setting: a cohort study in Indonesia. BMC Health Serv Res 2016;16(1):26.

36. Borg J, Lindström A, Larsson S. Assistive technology in developing countries: national and international responsibilities to implement the Convention on the Rights of Persons with Disabilities. Lancet 2009;374(9704):1863–5.

37. Tangcharoensathien V, Witthayapipopsakul W, Viriyathorn S, et al. Improving access to assistive technologies: challenges and solutions in low- and middle-income countries. WHO South East Asia J Public Health 2018;7(2):84–9.

38. Boisselle AK, Grajo LC. They Said: a global perspective on access to assistive technology. Open J Occup Ther 2018;6(3). https://doi.org/10.15453/2168-6408.1541.

39. Li W, Sellers C. Improving assistive technology economics for people with disabilities: Harnessing the voluntary and education sectors. In: 2009 IEEE Toronto International Conference Science and Technology for Humanity (TIC-STH). 2009. Toronto, Ontario, September 26–27, 2009.

40. Neumann PJ, Goldie SJ, Weinstein MC. Preference-based measures in economic evaluation in health care. Annu Rev Public Health 2000;21:587–611.

41. Brazier J. Measuring and valuing health benefits for economic evaluation. Oxford: Oxford University Press; 2007.

42. Morris S, Devlin N, Parkin D, et al. Economic analysis in healthcare. New Jersey: John Wiley & Sons; 2012.

43. Marasinghe KM, Lapitan JM, Ross A. Assistive technologies for ageing populations in six low-income and middle-income countries: a systematic review. BMJ Innov 2015;1(4):182–95.

44. Matter R, Harniss M, Oderud T, et al. Assistive technology in resource-limited environments: a scoping review. Disabil Rehabil Assist Technol 2017;12(2):105–14.

45. Instituto Nacional de Estadística y Censos. Incidencia de La Pobreza Y La Indigencia En 31 Aglomerados Urbanos. Ministerio de Hacienda. Available at: https://www.indec.gob.ar/uploads/informesdeprensa/eph_pobreza_01_18.pdf. Accessed October 16, 2018.

46. Instituto Nacional de Estadística y Censos (INDEC). Estudio Nacional Sobre El Perl de Las Personas Con Discapacidad: Resultados Preliminares 2018. Buenos Aires: Ministerio de Hacienda; 2018. Available at: https://www.indec.gov.ar/ftp/cuadros/poblacion/estudio_discapacidad_07_18.pdf. Accessed October 16, 2018.

47. Ley 25.504 Sistema de Protección integral de Los Discapacitados. 2001. Available at: http://servicios.infoleg.gob.ar/infolegInternet/anexos/70000-74999/70726/norma.htm. Accessed September 10, 2019.

48. Rossi C, Basset MN, Samman N. Estado nutricional de escolares y sus variables socioeconómicas. In: Encuentro Nacional de Nutricionistas AADYND. 2014. Available at: https://www.conicet.gov.ar/new_scp/detalle.php?keywords=&id=34046&congresos=yes&detalles=yes&congr_id=2362348. Accessed October 16, 2018.

49. World Health Organization, UNESCO, International Labour Organization & International Disability Development Consortium. 2010 Community-based rehabilitation: CBR guidelines. Available at: http://www.who.int/iris/handle/10665/44405. Accessed September 10, 2019.

50. Organization WH, Others. Wheelchair service training package–Basic level. Geneva (Switzerland): World Health Organization; 2017. p. 15.

51. Brazilian Institute of Geography and Statistics-IBGE. 2010 demographic census - General characteristics of the population, religion and people with disabilities 2010. Rio de Janeiro: Brazilian Institute of Geography and Statistics-IBGE.

52. World Health Organization. Rehabilitation in health systems 2017. Geneva (Switzerland). World Health Organization.

53. Presidencia da República. 2009 Decreto No 6.949. Promulga a Convenção Internacional sobre os Direitos das Pessoas com Deficiência e seu Protocolo Facultativo, assinados em Nova York, em 30 de março de 2007. Brasilia. Available at: http://www.planalto.gov.br/ccivil_03/_ato2007-2010/2009/decreto/d6949.htm. Accessed September 11, 2019.

54. Ribeiro CTM, Ribeiro MG, Araújo AP, et al. [The public health care system and rehabilitation actions in Brazil]. Rev Panam Salud Publica 2010;28(1):43–8.

55. Censo Nacional de Población y Vivienda. Segunda entrega preliminar 2018. Bogotá: Departamento Administrativo Nacional de Estadística; 2018. Available at: https://sitios.dane.gov.co/cnpv-presentacion/src/. Accessed November 26, 2018.

56. World Bank. Colombia country profile. World Bank. Available at: http://databank.worldbank.org/data/views/reports/reportwidget.aspx?Report_Name=CountryProfile&Id=b450fd57&tbar=y&dd=y&inf=n&zm=n&country=COL. Accessed October 1, 2018.

57. de Colombi G. Víctimas de Minas Antipersonal y Municiones sin Explosionar. Acción Contra Minas 2018. Available at: http://www.accioncontraminas.gov.co/estadisticas/Paginas/victimas-minas-antipersonal.aspx. Accessed October 1, 2018.

58. Agencia de la ONU para los Refugiados. Desplazamiento Forzado En 2017. United Nations. 2017. Available at: http://www.acnur.org/5b2956a04.pdf. Accessed September 10, 2019.

59. Asamble Nacional Constituyente. Constitución política de Colombia. 1991. Gaceta Constitucional No. 116 de 20 de julio de 1991.

60. Cifras de aseguramiento en salud. Ministerio de Salud y Protección Social. 2018. Available at: https://www.minsalud.gov.co/proteccionsocial/Paginas/cifras-aseguramiento-salud.aspx. Accessed August 10, 2018.

61. Vélez AL. La acción de tutela: ¿un mecanismo de protección del derecho a la salud y un proceso alterno para acceder a servicios de salud? Colomb Med 2005;36(3):199–208.

62. Ministerio de las Tecnologías de la Información y las Comunicaciones. Centro de Relevo. Centro de Relevo. Available at: https://centroderelevo.gov.co/632/w3-channel.html. Accessed October 23, 2018.

63. Congreso de Colombia. Ley 1145 de 2007: Por Medio de La Cual Se Organiza El Sistema Nacional de Discapacidad Y Se Dictan Otras Disposiciones. 2007. Available at: https://oig.cepal.org/sites/default/files/2007_ley1145_col.pdf. Accessed September 10, 2019.

64. Sentencia T-102. 2007. Available at: http://www.corteconstitucional.gov.co/relatoria/2007/T-102-07.htm. Accessed September 10, 2019.

65. Ministerio de Salud y Protección Social. Política Pública Nacional de Discapacidad E Inclusión Social 2013-2022. Bogotá 2014. Available at: https://www.minsalud.gov.co/sites/rid/Lists/BibliotecaDigital/RIDE/DE/PS/politica-publica-discapacidad-2013-2022.pdf. Accessed September 10, 2019.

66. Consejo Nacional de Política Económica y Social. Conpes social 166: Política Pública Nacional de Discapacidad E Inclusión Social. 2013. Available at: https://colaboracion.dnp.gov.co/cdt/conpes/social/166.pdf. Accessed September 10, 2019.

67. Lineamientos nacionales de rehabilitación basada en la comunidad - RBC. Bogotá: Ministerio de Salud y Protección Social. Available at: https://www.minsalud.gov.co/sites/rid/Lists/BibliotecaDigital/RIDE/VS/PP/ENT/lineamientos-nacionales-rbc.pdf

68. Cruz Velandia I, Fernández Moreno A, Duarte Cuervo C, et al. Sistematización de Investigaciones En Discapacidad Y En La Estrategia de Rehabilitación Basada En Comunidad (RBC). Bogotá DC Período 2005-2010. Alcaldía Mayor de Bogotá; 2014. Available at: http://repositoriocdpd.net:8080/handle/123456789/591.

69. Congreso de Colombia. Ley 1680 de 2013: Por La Cual Se Garantiza a Las Personas Ciegas Y Con Baja Visión, El Acceso a La Información, a Las Comunicaciones, Al Conocimiento Y a Las Tecnologías de La Información Y de Las Comunicaciones. Available at: http://www.secretariasenado.gov.co/senado/basedoc/ley_1680_2013.html. Accessed September 10, 2019.

70. Inicio - ConVerTic. Available at: http://www.convertic.gov.co/641/w3-channel.html. Accessed August 23, 2018.

71. Ministerio de Salud y Protección Social. Resolución 5592 de 2015. 2015. p. 220. Available at: https://www.minsalud.gov.co/Normatividad_Nuevo/Resoluci%C3%B3n%205592%20de%202015.pdf. Accessed September 10, 2019.

72. Congreso de Colombia. Ley 1751 de 2015: Por Medio de La Cual Se Regula El Derecho Fundamental a La Salud Y Se Dictan Otras Disposiciones 2015. Available at: https://www.minsalud.gov.co/Normatividad_Nuevo/Ley%201751%20de%202015.pdf. Accessed September 10, 2019.

73. Ministerio de Salud y Protección Social. ABECÉ de la Discapacidad 2014. Available at: https://www.minsalud.gov.co/sites/rid/Lists/BibliotecaDigital/RIDE/DE/PS/abece-de-la-discapacidad.pdf. Accessed September 10, 2019.

74. Ministerio de Salud y Protección Social. Resolución 2968 de 2015: Por La Cual Se Establecen Los Requisitos Sanitarios Que Deben Cumplir Los Establecimientos Que Elaboran Y Adaptan Dispositivos Médicos Sobre Medida de Tecnología Ortopédica Externa Ubicados En El Territorio Nacional. p. 16. Available at: https://paginaweb.invima.gov.co/images/pdf/normatividad/dispositivos-medicos/resoluciones/Resolución%202968%20de%202015.pdf. Accessed September 10, 2019.

75. Ministerio de Salud y Protección Social. Resolución 5267 de 2017 2017. Available at: https://www.minsalud.gov.co/sites/rid/Lists/BibliotecaDigital/RIDE/DE/DIJ/resolucion-5267-de-2017.pdf. Accessed September 10, 2019.

76. de Sanidad Militar DG. Protocolo Administrativo Para La Prescripción, Seguimiento Y Control de Los Productos de Apoyo En Salud Para El SSFM. Bogotá: Ministerio de Defensa Nacional; 2015.

77. Resolución 350 de 2016: Por Medio de La Cual Se Reglamentan La Implementación de Los Sistemas de Acceso En Los Contenidos Transmitidos a Través Del Servicio Público de Televisión Que Garantizan El Acceso de Las Personas Con Discapacidad Auditiva Y Se Dictan Otras Disposiciones. Available at: https://www.icbf.gov.co/cargues/avance/docs/resolucion_antv_0350_2016.htm. Accessed October 24, 2018.

78. Ministerio de Educación Nacional. Decreto 1421 de 2017: Por El Cual Se Reglamenta En El Marco de La Educación Inclusiva La Atención Educativa a La Población Con Discapacidad 2017. p. 20. Available at: http://es.presidencia.gov.co/normativa/normativa/DECRETO%201421%20DEL%2029%20DE%20AGOSTO%20DE%202017.pdf. Accessed September 10, 2019.

79. Ministerio de Educación Nacional. Guía Para La Implementación Del Decreto 1421 de 2017. Bogotá: Ministerio de Eudcación; 2018. Available at: http://aprende.colombiaaprende.edu.co/ckfinder/userfiles/files/Guia%20de%20apoyo%20-%20Decreto%201421%20de%202017%2016022018%20(1).pdf.

80. de Colombia G. Bienvenido a Biblioteca Virtual para Ciegos de Colombia | Biblioteca Virtual para Ciegos de Colombia. Instituto Nacional Para Ciegos INCI. Available at: http://biblioteca.inci.gov.co/. Accessed October 24, 2018.

81. Ministerio de Trabajo. Decreto 2011 de 2017. p. 4. Available at: http://es.presidencia.gov.co/normativa/normativa/DECRETO%202011%20DEL%2030%20DE%20NOVIEMBRE%20DE%202017.pdf. Accessed September 10, 2019.

82. Lucas Correa-Montoya JCR-SMV-I. #EscuelaParaTodos: Panorama Y Retos Del Derecho a La Educación Inclusiva de Las Personas Con Discapacidad En Colombia. Bogotá: DescLAB; 2018. Available at: https://www.desclab.com/educacion-inclusiva. Accessed August 24, 2018.

83. Rehabilitación física. Comité Internacional de la Cruz Roja. Available at: https://www.icrc.org/es/nuestras-actividades/salud/rehabilitacion-fisica. Accessed October 1, 2018.

84. Humanity and Inclusion Colombi. ¿Quiénes somos?. Available at: http://humanityandinclusioncolombia.com/quienes-somos/. Accessed October 1, 2018.

85. Concha FS. Proyecto TEAM: transformando vidas. Fundación Saldarriaga Concha 2018. Available at: https://saldarriagaconcha.org/desarrollo_fsc/es/fsc-como-trabajamos/item/955-proyecto-team-transformando-vidas. Accessed October 24, 2018.

86. Coaliación Colombiana por la Implementación de la Convención sobre los Derechos de las Personas con Discapacidad. Available at: https://discapacidadcolombia.com/phocadownloadpap/PUBLICACIONES_ARTICULOS/Informe%20Alterno%20Coalicion%20Colombiana%20-%20esp.pdf. Accessed September 10, 2019.

87. Montoya C, Lucas Y, Martínez C, et al. Discapacidad E Inclusión Social En Colombia. Informe Alternativo de La Fundación Saldarriaga Concha Al Comité de Naciones Unidas Sobre Los Derechos de Las Personas Con Discapacidad. Editorial Fundación Saldarriaga Concha 2016. Available at: https://saldarriagaconcha.

org/desarrollo_fsc/images/Informe_Alternativo_campa%C3%B1a.pdf. Accessed September 10, 2019.

88. Mishra S, DeMuth S, Sabharwal S, et al. Disability and rehabilitation in Tajikistan: development of a multisectoral national programme to leave no one behind. Public health panorama 2018;4(2):202–9.

89. Ministry of Social Justice and Empowerment. ALIMCO signed ToT agreement with motivation charitable trust of U.K to manufacture WHO compliant wheelchairs in India 2016. Government of India. Press Information Bureau. Available at: https://pib.gov.in/newsite/PrintRelease.aspx?relid=155700. Accessed September 10, 2019.

90. Hamner SR, Narayan VG, Donaldson KM. Designing for scale: development of the ReMotion Knee for global emerging markets. Ann Biomed Eng 2013;41(9): 1851–9.

91. International Society of Wheelchair Professionals Policy Advocacy Toolkit. Available at: http://pak.wheelchairnetwork.org. Accessed September 10, 2019.

92. Frehywot S, Vovides Y, Talib Z, et al. E-learning in medical education in resource constrained low- and middle-income countries. Hum Resour Health 2013;11:4.

93. Liyanagunawardena TR, Aboshady OA. Massive open online courses: a resource for health education in developing countries. Glob Health Promot 2018;25(3):74–6.

94. WHO. Priority assistive products list (APL) 2017. Available at: http://www.who.int/phi/implementation/assistive_technology/global_survey-apl/en/. Accessed September 4, 2018.

95. Wheelchair International Network – Training management system for the wheelchair sector. Available at: http://wheelchairnetwork.org/. Accessed September 4, 2018.

96. News & Press. Available at: https://www.ispoint.org/page/Accreditation. Accessed September 4, 2018.

97. CECOPS. Available at: http://www.cecops.org.uk/. Accessed September 4, 2018.

98. Market Shaping Primer. Available at: https://www.usaid.gov/cii/market-shaping-primer. Accessed August 30, 2018.

99. Lin A, Wilson J. Healthy markets for global health: a market shaping primer. Washington, DC: Center for Accelerating Innovation and Impact, United States Agency for International Development; 2014. p. 2018.

100. Home. ATscale. Available at: https://atscale2030.org. Accessed August 30, 2018.

Facilitators and Barriers to the Rehabilitation Workforce Capacity Building in Low- to Middle-Income Countries

Amaramalar Selvi Naicker, MBBS, M. Rehab Med., CIME[a],*,
Ohnmar Htwe, MBBS, MMedSc (Rehab Med), CMIA[a],
Abena Yeboaa Tannor, BSc, MBChB, MSc (Rehab), MGCP[b],
Wouter De Groote, MD, PMR, Post Grad Rehabilitation Management in LMIC[c,1],
Brenda Saria Yuliawiratman, MBBS, M. Rehab Med, CMIA[a],
Manimalar Selvi Naicker, MBBS, MPath, MMedStats[d]

KEYWORDS

• Rehabilitation • Low middle income • Capacity building • Various • Facilitators
• Barriers

KEY POINTS

- An estimated increase in population and chronic conditions leading to disability required increasing emphasis on rehabilitation and fundamental health intervention.
- Unlike developed nations, the poorer countries do not usually have the full rehabilitation workforce needed to promote societal inclusion and participation while improving quality of life.
- In general, roles/job scope of rehabilitation workforce was not clearly defined and often resorted to task shifting, thus leading to more barriers and facilitators in capacity building.
- Barriers were poor availability of human resources and insufficient training program/supports for their professional development. Facilitators were local government support and international non-governmental organizations collaboration.
- Recommendations for capacity building effort are to work together with the developed nations to encourage funding, training, education, and sharing of resources.

Disclosure Statement: The authors have nothing to disclose.
[a] Rehabilitation Medicine Unit, Department of Orthopedics and Traumatology, Faculty of Medicine, University Kebangsaan Malaysia, Jalan Yaacob Latif, Bandar Tun Razak, Cheras, Kuala Lumpur 56000, Malaysia; [b] Department of Family Medicine, Komfo Anokye Teaching Hospital, Kwame Nkrumah University of Science and Technology, PO EBox 1934, Kumasi, Ghana; [c] Department of Rehabilitation Medicine, St Jozef, Bornem, Belgium; [d] Department of Pathology, Faculty of Medicine, University of Malaya, Kuala Lumpur 50603, Malaysia
[1] Present address: Kruisabeelstraat 124, Moorsel 9310, Belgium.
* Corresponding author.
E-mail address: asnaicker@yahoo.com

Phys Med Rehabil Clin N Am 30 (2019) 867–877
https://doi.org/10.1016/j.pmr.2019.07.009
pmr.theclinics.com

INTRODUCTION

Fifteen percent of the world's population, according to the World Health Organization (WHO), is known to have some form of disability. Eighty percent of them are in low- to middle-income countries (LMIC) with an unforgiving cycle of poverty and disability. The estimated increase in population is likely to lead to chronic conditions and disabilities.[1] Persons with disabilities (PWD) deserve rehabilitation, a fundamental health intervention, which is promoted by the WHO Rehabilitation 2030 initiative.

An ideal multidisciplinary team is crucial to optimize the function, independence, and quality of life of PWD. It consists of rehabilitation physicians, nurses, physical and occupational therapists (OTs), speech and language therapists, orthotists, and prosthetists who play important roles in the lives of PWD both in hospitals and in the communities. Hospital roles include initial assessments, diagnoses, and provision of inpatient rehabilitation as well as psychological support, patient, and family education.[2] Thus, the rehabilitation workforce serves to promote societal inclusion and participation while improving the quality of life of PWD into the community.[3]

There is a dearth of rehabilitation professionals in LMIC compared with high-income countries (HIC) with very little to no training institutions. The WHO's Rehabilitation 2030 Call for Action agenda noted that there are insufficient numbers of rehabilitation professionals, almost one-tenth of that required, and a density of less than 10 per million for skilled practitioners.[4] The WHO's Global Disability Action Plan 2015 to 2021 also noted one of the barriers experienced by PWD to be lack of service provision,[1] which negatively impacts PWD.

The 2006 United Nations Convention on the Rights of Persons with Disabilities articles[5–7] had tasked members to organize and provide training for health professionals in order to improve access to rehabilitation services for PWD, and WHO in 2015 urged states to "Produce national standards in training for different types and levels of rehabilitation and habilitation personnel that can enable career development and continuing education across levels."[1,8]

The International Society of Physical and Rehabilitation Medicine (ISPRM) is a non-governmental organization (NGO) serving as the international umbrella organization for rehabilitation physicians and the WHO's collaborator on disability and rehabilitation issues.[9]

As part of liaising activities with the WHO, ISPRM during its 10th World Congress in Malaysia commissioned its working group on capacity building of the rehabilitation workforce in LMIC with the aim to unearth the facilitators and barriers to the rehabilitation workforce capacity building in LMIC.

This report thus presents findings of the working group via a systematic review.

Goals of the working group were to identify facilitators and barriers to the capacity building of rehabilitation workforce in LMIC as well as provide recommendations and strategies needed for the process.

METHODOLOGY

The technical team of the ISPRM-WHO Working Group for this project comprised rehabilitation physicians from Malaysia, Ghana, and Belgium. The search strategy in later discussion was used for the literature search.

Search Strategy

Databases searched: Medline, PubMed, CINHAL, and Cochrane Database
Database Host: National Library of Medicine, EBSCOHOST, Cochrane Library

Other searches: Google, Google Scholar

Date search was run: June 2017

Years covered by search: No restrictions

Complete search strategy: Search (rehab*) OR/AND ((LMIC) OR poor country) OR (developing county) OR (low resource country) AND ((rich country) OR HIC) OR (MIC)

Summary of the search strategy: Related to health condition or intervention: rehabilitation, team development, capacity building, developing countries, Africa, facilitators, barriers, challenges. Related to study design: Not specified.

Hand searching: Secondary literature search from reference list of e-searched articles

Gray literature: Centre for International Rehabilitation Information and Exchange Database of International Rehabilitation Research

Restrictions: Restricted to English language and human studies

Project discussions and communications were via e-mail and Skype meetings, and the group worked to put together the collective data and write up this article.

RESULTS

The searches produced 32 papers, of which full-text reports were acquired. The reviewers then selected 19 papers based on relevance and closeness to the objectives. The papers consisted of 5 descriptive papers,[10–14] 6 review articles,[5,7,15–18] 5 qualitative research papers,[19–23] 1 theoretic model,[6] 1 cross-sectional study,[24] and 1 paper that is part of an education project of the Global Health Education Consortium.[2]

The papers looked at various aspects of perception of rehabilitation professionals, experiences with service delivery, competencies, and availability of rehabilitation workforce, prevalence of impairment, accessibility and challenges in implementing rehabilitation services, as well as coping skills of rehabilitation professionals in various LMIC settings. Others explored rehabilitation needs, training, and education among their existing workforce. Based on **Table 1**, several issues can be highlighted on barriers and facilitators in capacity building of rehabilitation workforce in low-resource countries.

Capacity Building of Rehabilitation Workforce

Some of the papers generally referred to the rehabilitation workforce, and thus, members and their roles were not clearly stated.[5,10,11,17,25] The rest of them had only 2 to 3 of the ideal rehabilitation team. A few papers mentioned community health/disability workers as well as physiotherapist (PT)/OT assistants whose job scopes were not clearly described.[7,11,19] In some instances, family physicians took on the role of rehabilitation doctors,[15,21] and much of the job scope was shared among available rehabilitation workers in various capacities (task shifting).

Support and training initiatives toward capacity building came from international as well as national agencies, government as well as NGOs.[6,10–12,14–16,18,19,21,25]

Barriers

Human resources and training

A shortage of rehabilitation physicians and allied health workers, lack of training programs for their professional development, absent or variable credentials, and/or licensing and lack of paid positions were among the challenges.

Variations in competencies, education, credentials, and typical practices, lack of adequate staff for physiotherapy training in universities, limited opportunities for

Table 1 Summary of the review	
Reference Number	**Summary**
Flett & Biggs,[5] 1993	Flett and colleagues looked at the coping skills of rehabilitation practitioners Facilitators: Women possess better coping skills than men and seek social support when necessary
Jesus et al,[6] 2016	Jesus and colleagues reported that facilitator was international exchange programs Barriers: Brain drain for greater economic opportunities, poor access to rehabilitation services, shortage of rehabilitation workers, unmet needs for physical therapy, centrally located physical therapist services, limited training center, lowest ratio of PT in Bangladesh (0.1 PT per 10,000 people), lack of funding or stakeholders' awareness, escalating chronic disabling condition
Jesus et al,[7] 2017	Jesus and colleagues highlighted that facilitators were in existence for long-distant education and international clinical education Barriers: Unstructured credentialing or licensing, variations in competencies, lack of training programs & staff, poor access to public transport, poor insurance coverage/uninsured for the poor in rural areas, lack of funding or stakeholders' awareness, poor government support, premature discharge from the ward irrespective of the recovery, inadequate equipment
Andrianabela et al,[10] 2015	Andrianabela and colleagues described a training program (Diploma) of rehabilitation doctors in Madagascar with the support of National Health Service (NHS) (UK) doctors Facilitators: The Diploma program was conducted with the faculty support of NHS (UK) doctors Barriers: The Diploma program was delayed by political instability, poor access to rehabilitation services and workers, limited facilities, funding
Khan et al,[11] 2015	Khan and colleagues looked at the challenges in implementing the WHO Disability Action Plan in Madagascar among general practitioners, PT, doctor, community health workers Facilitators: Political commitment to improving care and support for person with disability (PWD) Barriers: Lack of available rehabilitation services and poor integration with acute health care systems, lack of infrastructure and IT support, poor geographic coverage, shortage of strong leadership and skilled workforce, poor awareness, cultural stigma
Vlak et al,[12] 2014	Vlak and colleagues looked at recent changes in rehabilitation medicine education universities in Croatia among rehabilitation doctors, PT Facilitators: Ministry of Health accreditation for young physical and rehabilitation medicine (PRM) physicians, inclusion of Rehabilitation Medicine in medical undergraduate training, establishing Rehabilitation Medicine training centers; Croatia: Second highest ratio of PRM specialists per 100,000 inhabitants among European Union Barriers: Rheumatology-based training for PRM specialists in Croatia, inadequate staff for physiotherapy training in universities
Rathore et al,[13] 2008	Rathore and colleagues described spinal cord injury rehabilitation report on earthquake in Pakistan (2005), including rehabilitation doctors, PT, OT, psychiatrists, & psychologists Facilitators: Established Armed Forces Institute of Rehabilitation Medicine in Pakistan (2005) Barriers: Inadequate rehabilitation specialists and training centers, lack of awareness by governments, health bureaucrats, or health professionals

(continued on next page)

Reference Number	Summary
O'Connell & Ingersoll A,[14] 2012	O'Connell and colleagues looked at upper-limb prosthetic services in Haiti after disaster among prosthetists & orthotists (P&O) Facilitators: Credentialed training program for P&O through Don Bosco University, El Salvador–Handicap International, expatriate assistance for training local staff Barriers: Natural disasters: Earthquake, shortage of trained P&O staff, inadequate local resources
Gupta et al,[15] 2011	Gupta and colleagues highlighted human resources for rehabilitation with cross-national findings of supply and need for rehabilitative personnel within and across regions among caregivers, PT, OT, speech language pathologist (SLP), P&O, family physician, wheelchair technician, nurses Facilitators: Utilization of CBR to make up for the shortage of rehabilitation professionals in some countries
Schiappacasse et al,[16] 2014	Schiappacasse and colleagues presented a report that reflects the 2003 National Survey of PWD by the government of Argentina, which looked at the prevalence of impairments that affected functions of everyday life in PWD and factors affecting their functional outcome Facilitators: Establishment of legislation that enhanced new laws and policies that mandate the establishment of a system of basic services in enabling rehabilitation for PWD, government's commitment to facilitate social integration of PWD by providing Certificate of Disability (UCD), 127 training institutes for PMR within Argentina Barriers: Poor labor force participation by PWD, poor access to public transport, poor policy implementation, poor housing conditions: not disabled friendly, shortage of skilled workforce, poor involvement of PRM societies in discussion of disability legislations
Shanmugasegaram et al,[17] 2014	Shanmugasegaram and colleagues reported "Accessibility and structure cardiac rehabilitation services (CRS) and the patients' outcomes in LMIC" among cardiac rehabilitation team Facilitators: Latin American programs offered multidisciplinary services led by the physicians, basic CR programs, for example,; tai chi Barriers: Lack of trained personnel for CRS and structured program, lack of perceived benefit or profitability, limited budget & dedicated space, inefficient public transport, inadequate insurance coverage for the poor in rural areas
Yousafzai et al,[18] 2014	Yousafzai and colleagues reported that considerable progress has been made over the last decade in recognizing the significant numbers of children with disability globally, and the associated risks and consequences for life outcomes Facilitators: National surveys on childhood disability, international agreements, such as the United Nations Convention on the Rights of Persons with Disabilities with the International Classification of Functioning, and CBR programs Barriers: Erratic training of CBR workers, insufficient training and awareness, families with poor knowledge, limited professional and government support, inadequate funding and available services
Lorenzo et al,[19] 2015	Lorenzo and colleagues reported on "Competencies of community disability workers (CDWs) in 3 southern African countries" Facilitators: Government support with training of CDWs who can educate primary health care workers Barriers: CDW in rural areas was often cross-disciplinary, limited opportunities, and lack of structured continuing professional development (CPD) programs

(continued on next page)

Table 1 (continued)	
Reference Number	**Summary**
Magnusson & Ramstrand,[20] 2009	Magnusson and colleagues looked at "Exploration of education in Pakistan Institute of Prosthetic & Orthotic Science" Facilitators: Established category II training center Barriers: Brain drain, poor upgrading of teachers' knowledge, limited opportunities for CPD and information technology, limited awareness by peers and general community, natural disaster interfering clinical training program
Mohd Nordin et al,[21] 2014	Nordin and colleagues looked at "Perception of rehabilitation professionals and stroke survivors toward long-term stroke rehabilitation services and potential approaches" among PT, OT, SLP, social worker, family physician Facilitators: Increasing support and awareness for poststroke rehabilitation within government hospitals Barriers: Lack of stakeholders' awareness, shortage of skilled workforces, limited funding, training center, access to rehabilitation services, public transport, and costly private services, lack of continuity of care and dedicated wards for stroke rehabilitation in government hospitals, poor patients/family involvement
Geere et al,[22] 2013	Geere and colleagues reported facilitators were training CBR workers by PT, enthusiastic caregivers who enable their children to attend school to create respite or opportunities for them to engage with other work, resilient and optimistic caregivers Barriers: Need of health care professionals' knowledge and skill in managing musculoskeletal pain, limited funding, clients' participation in therapy that eventually impacts on therapist motivation to practice, emotional aspect of caregivers and their spinal pain, equipment, and logistic issues
Harms & Kobusingye,[23] 2003	Harms and Kobusingye reported that facilitators were modification of programs and plans for CBR, motivated caregivers, patients' trust in professionals, poor access to public transport, cost of transport, interruption of employment, and lost income Barriers: The lengthy waiting time to have assistive devices or the cost, unaware of rehabilitation services by other health care professionals because the rehabilitation profession is relatively new in Uganda, unfamiliar with physiotherapy and lack of awareness of the therapy, strong belief in traditional healers or bonesetters (major barrier)
Christian et al,[24] 2011	Christian and colleagues reported "Rehabilitation needs and services postdischarge from an African trauma center" among PT Facilitators: Good trauma centers in Ghana Barriers: Poor research on the need for PRM, lack of awareness on the need for rehabilitation workforce
Pechak & Thompson,[25] 2007	Pechak and Thompson reported "Part of an Education project of the global health education consortium" among rehabilitation workforce Facilitators: Developed and developing countries universities' collaboration, educational resources for training, especially CBR workers Barriers: Brain drain for greater economic opportunities, absence of or variable credentials or licensing, lack of paid positions, erratic training of CBR workers

continuing professional development, and support for community disability workers led to poor professional recognition and training.[4,6,7,9,10,13,16,17,19,21]

Inadequate availability of rehabilitation equipment and material supplies contributed significantly to these challenges.[7,14]

Governmental and policy implementation

The poor governmental support manifested as a lack of insurance coverage for staff, especially those in remote areas, and lack of leadership in providing standard rehabilitation care in government hospitals. Furthermore, lack of awareness on the need for rehabilitation on the part of government, bureaucrats, and health professional was a stumbling block in capacity building among the rehabilitation workforce. Poor policy implementation and inadequate reported data resulted in a shortage of services in inland areas. Other causes include poor research on the need for rehabilitation and lack of funding and stakeholder awareness.[6,7,9–13,15,16,18,21,24]

The availability and use of quality, comparable data, and information within and across countries are needed to support human resources for strategy development, rehabilitation policy, and practice.

Client and caregiver perspectives

Lack of emphasis on emotional well-being and health of the caregivers led to the lack of parental cooperation.[22] The caregivers were often not participatory owing to the lack of confidence, awareness and time,[21] and complaints of back pain, which calls for a strong need for health care professionals to improve their knowledge and skill in managing musculoskeletal pain.[14] From the consumer's viewpoint, unfamiliarity with the need for therapy, demotivation, a stronger belief toward traditional healers and bone setters,[10,23] undesirable cultural stigma, and poor awareness about disabilities and rehabilitation were among the challenges faced.[11]

Geopolitical

Geopolitical instability was also cited as a significant barrier in capacity building in LMIC.[8,14] Poor public transport along with the exorbitant cost and inadequate geographic coverage made logistics a significant barrier for rehabilitation staff wanting to carry out their tasks.[7,11,16,17,21,23]

Facilitators

Some significant facilitators were also observed in this review. A few LMIC received help in the form of faculty support, credential training program, university, and international NGOs collaborations.[10,14,25] The local government support was present in various capacities, such as provision of educational resources, international exchange programs, and long-distance educational and clinical service placement. With some countries enforcing legislation toward enabling a comprehensive rehabilitation for PWD,[6,11,16,18] political commitment to improve care and support for PWD can be perceived. In fact, since 2005, Croatia took significant steps to support rehabilitation medicine education and training for young physicians.[12] Some African countries had their governments supporting the training of community disability workers[19](see Table 1).

DISCUSSION

This research project under the auspices of the ISPRM-WHO working group was undertaken across countries by several dedicated and experienced rehabilitation physicians who contributed to the capacity building of rehabilitation personnel in LMIC settings. Only a limited amount of articles was found related to the subject of barriers and facilitators. Challenges faced in reviewing articles related to the project were limited studies on capacity building of the rehabilitation workforces and this may have been due to:

- Variable levels of resources and infrastructure are available for the training of rehabilitation workers and delivering services.
- Building and equipping medical rehabilitation institutions and training professional rehabilitation personnel are not a realistic solution for all countries and settings.
- There are different levels of education, work scope, and practice patterns among rehabilitation professionals.
- Rehabilitation professionals emigrate to HIC to seek greater economic opportunities.

The rehabilitation workforce was incomplete, whereas the job scope was also shared (task shifting). Much of the support and training came from international and national NGOs.

At the organizational level, the health system structure, policies, and procedures should be tailored to the needs of health care providers, professionals, and end users. At the individual level, optimization of skills, experience, and knowledge of rehabilitation is crucial. Fellowship exchange programs, scholarship programs, and basic and advanced training programs are among the interventions that are important.[26]

Poor availability of human resources, lack of training program, and poor governmental support, that is inadequate policy implementation and initiative in providing standard rehabilitation care, were significant barriers. Challenges were also faced from the caregivers and clients who were often not participatory because of a lack of confidence, awareness, time, and undesirable culture stigma.

Geopolitical instability and poor availability of the infrastructure also contributed barriers for capacity building of the rehabilitation personnel.

Assistance from local government through the provision of educational supports, international exchange programs, screening services, and clinical service placement as well as political will and commitment in enforcing legislation were significant contributors.

Committed politicians, effective managers, motivated workers, effective institutions, and involved communities can take many constructive steps, even in difficult financial circumstances.

In order to support more effective systems, community-based rehabilitation (CBR) and disability activists should seek to build capacity with skilled individuals who are supported by strong organizations which might be at the local, regional, or country levels.

Policies must be responsive to the needs and social values of people with disabilities. Sustainable change also depends on organizations learning lessons over time; they need an institutional memory that helps them focus regardless of changing priorities.[27]

SUMMARY AND RECOMMENDATIONS

Although LMIC may be challenged in facilitating capacity building in comparison to more HIC, working together to assist in the form of funding, training, and education as well as sharing resources and practice by more developed nations can greatly improve rehabilitation outcome while also improving on building capacity within the rehabilitation workforce in LMIC nations. In the long run, all capacity building efforts should be local and institutionalized.

Recommendations

Based on the research, strategic recommendations have been made and grouped under 3 themes: training, evaluation, and support. These recommendations are to assist LMIC and ISPRM in achieving WHO's goal of capacity building of the rehabilitation workforce in LMIC.

Training
1. Organization of frequent continuous professional development workshops for the rehabilitation workforce in their specific fields of work. These workshops should be tailored to expertise and skills in academic, research, administrative, financial, managerial, and diverse technical and nontechnical fields essential for delivering optimum service.
2. Facilitating collaborations between local rehabilitation professionals and external well-established professionals for mentorship and professional exchange programs.
3. Establishment of coordinated telemedicine training using simple technology, such as mobile phones for rehabilitation consultations.
4. Development and delivery of additional technology-assisted education modules (eg, mobile apps).
5. Establishment of in-country and internationally standardized curricula for professional training of underrepresented workforce members, for example, OT, community rehabilitation workers.

Evaluation
6. Facilitating the use of external/foreign professional examiners in skills evaluation of rehabilitation professionals in order to maintain a high standard of training.
7. Use of service delivery evaluation tools (Rehabilitation Management System, WHO Rehabilitation Support Package) and organization of visits by experts to rehabilitation centers to evaluate rehabilitation service delivery.
8. Conducting original scientific rehabilitation workforce capacity research, reviews, and outcomes of capacity building.

Support
9. Increasing awareness to policymakers in LMIC on the importance of coordinated multidisciplinary medical rehabilitation services. Policymakers should be well informed about the increasing demand of rehabilitation services in their countries as noncommunicable diseases become more prevalent, and the need to allocate adequate budgetary resources to building capacity and service.
10. Public awareness creation about the benefits of medical rehabilitation.
11. Marketing of the different rehabilitation workforce professions in order to increase enrollment in training programs.
12. Institution of educational grants and scholarships for the training of rehabilitation professionals.
13. Early placement on salary scales after training, and challenging career opportunities.
14. Facilitating the in-country curriculum tailored to the needs of rehabilitation professionals and clients in LMIC.
15. Institutional support for leadership.
16. Establishment of professional bodies for all rehabilitation personnel in LMIC.

STUDY LIMITATIONS

Most of the papers dealt with barriers on rehabilitation services rather than challenges in capacity building of rehabilitation work force. The papers also did not define clearly the roles of the rehabilitation members wherein ill-defined terms of reference, such as therapists, community health workers, and community disability workers, were used. Furthermore, varying methodological designs were used, making meaningful comparison challenging. Many of the papers were qualitative with no fixed outcome measures.

ACKNOWLEDGMENTS

General research facilities were provided by University Kebangsaan Malaysia, University of Malaya, and Komfo Anokye Teaching Hospital.

REFERENCES

1. World Health Organization. WHO global disability action plan 2014-2021: Better health for all people with disability. Geneva (Switzerland): World Health Organization; 2014.
2. Momsen AM, Rasmussen JO, Nielsen CV, et al. Multidisciplinary team care in rehabilitation: an overview of reviews. J Rehabil Med 2012;44(11):901–12.
3. World Health Organization. Community-based rehabilitation: CBR guidelines. 2010. Available at: http://www.who.int/disabilities/cbr/guidelines/en/index.html. Accessed October 30, 2017.
4. World Health Organization. Rehabilitation 2030: the need to scale up rehabilitation. Geneva (Switzerland): World Health Organization; 2017.
5. Flett R, Biggs H. Wellbeing and the rehabilitation service provider: the role of coping strategies. Int J Rehabil Res 1993;16(4):313–5.
6. Jesus TS, Koh G, Landry M, et al. Finding the "right-size" physical therapy workforce: international perspective across 4 countries. Phys Ther 2016;96(10): 1597–609.
7. Jesus TS, Landry MD, Dussault G, et al. Human resources for health (and rehabilitation): six rehab-workforce challenges for the century. Hum Resour Health 2017;15:8.
8. Convention on the Rights of Persons with Disabilities. New York: United Nations; 2007. Available at: https:/www.un.org/disabilities/document/convention.
9. Stucki G, Reinhardt JD, Imamura M, et al. Developing the International Society of Physical and Rehabilitation Medicine (ISPRM): following through. J Rehabil Med 2011;43(1):1–7.
10. Andrianabela S, Hariharan R, Ford HL, et al. A rehabilitation training partnership in Madagascar. J Rehabil Med 2015;47(8):682–7.
11. Khan F, Amatya B, Mannan H, et al. Rehabilitation in Madagascar: challenges in implementing the World Health Organization disability action plan. J Rehabil Med 2015;47(8):688–96.
12. Vlak T, Soso D, Poljicanin A, et al. Physical and rehabilitation medicine training center in Split, Croatia: striving to achieve excellence in education of a rehabilitation team. Disabil Rehabil 2014;36(9):781–6.
13. Rathore FA, Farooq F, Muzammil S, et al. Spinal cord injury management and rehabilitation: highlights and shortcomings from the 2005 earthquake in Pakistan. Arch Phys Med Rehabil 2008;89(3):579–85.

14. O'Connell C, Ingersoll A. Upper limb prosthetic services post Haiti earthquake: experiences and recommendations of Haiti-based rehabilitation program. J Prosthet Orthot 2012;24(2):77–9.
15. Gupta N, Castillo-Laborde C, Landry MD. Health-related rehabilitation services: assessing the global supply of and need for human resources. BMC Health Serv Res 2011;11:276.
16. Schiappacasse C, Longoni M, Paleo MA, et al. Reflecting on the world report on disability: a short report from Argentina. Am J Phys Med Rehabil 2014;93(1 Suppl 1):S39–41.
17. Shanmugasegaram S, Perez-Terzic C, Jiang X, et al. Cardiac rehabilitation services in low- and middle-income countries: a scoping review. J Cardiovasc Nurs 2014;29(5):454–63.
18. Yousafzai AK, Lynch P, Gladstone M. Moving beyond prevalence studies: screening and interventions for children with disabilities in low-income and middle-income countries. Arch Dis Child 2014;99(9):840–8.
19. Lorenzo T, van Pletzen E, Booyens M. Determining the competences of community based workers for disability-inclusive development in rural areas of South Africa, Botswana and Malawi. Rural Remote Health 2015;15(2):2919.
20. Magnusson L, Ramstrand N. Prosthetist/orthotist educational experience & professional development in Pakistan. Disabil Rehabil Assist Technol 2009;4(6):385–92.
21. Mohd Nordin NA, Aziz NA, Abdul Aziz AF, et al. Exploring views on long term rehabilitation for people with stroke in a developing country: findings from focus group discussions. BMC Health Serv Res 2014;14:118.
22. Geere JL, Gona J, Omondi FO, et al. Caring for children with physical disability in Kenya: potential links between caregiving and carers' physical health. Child Care Health Dev 2013;39(3):381–92.
23. Harms S, Kobusingye O. Factors that influence the use of rehabilitation services in an urban Ugandan hospital. Int J Rehabil Res 2003;26(1):73–7.
24. Christian A, Gonzalez-Fernandez M, Mayer RS, et al. Rehabilitation needs of persons discharged from an African trauma center. Pan Afr Med J 2011;10:32.
25. Pechak C, Thompson M. Disability and Rehabilitation in Developing Countries. An education project of the Global Health Education Consortium. Global Health Course Modules Project 2007.
26. Capacity building: United Nation Development Program (UNDP) Primer paper. In: Wignaraja K, editor. New York: United Nations Development Programme; 2009. Available at: www.undp.org/capacity.
27. Kuipers P. Improving disability and rehabilitation systems in low and middle-income countries: some lessons from health systems strengthening. Disability, CBR and Inclusive Development Journal 2014;25(2):90–6.

UNITED STATES POSTAL SERVICE ®

Statement of Ownership, Management, and Circulation
(All Periodicals Publications Except Requester Publications)

1. Publication Title
PHYSICAL MEDICINE AND REHABILITATION CLINICS OF NORTH AMERICA

2. Publication Number
009 – 243

3. Filing Date
9/18/2019

4. Issue Frequency
FEB, MAY, AUG, NOV

5. Number of Issues Published Annually
4

6. Annual Subscription Price
$304.00

7. Complete Mailing Address of Known Office of Publication (Not printer) (Street, city, county, state, and ZIP+4®)
ELSEVIER INC.
230 Park Avenue, Suite 800
New York, NY 10169

Contact Person
STEPHEN R. BUSHING

Telephone (Include area code)
215-239-3688

8. Complete Mailing Address of Headquarters or General Business Office of Publisher (Not printer)
ELSEVIER INC.
230 Park Avenue, Suite 800
New York, NY 10169

9. Full Names and Complete Mailing Addresses of Publisher, Editor, and Managing Editor (Do not leave blank)

Publisher (Name and complete mailing address)
TAYLOR BALL, ELSEVIER INC.
1600 JOHN F KENNEDY BLVD. SUITE 1800
PHILADELPHIA, PA 19103-2899

Editor (Name and complete mailing address)
LAUREN BOYLE, ELSEVIER INC.
1600 JOHN F KENNEDY BLVD. SUITE 1800
PHILADELPHIA, PA 19103-2899

Managing Editor (Name and complete mailing address)
PATRICK MANLEY, ELSEVIER INC.
1600 JOHN F KENNEDY BLVD. SUITE 1800
PHILADELPHIA, PA 19103-2899

10. Owner (Do not leave blank. If the publication is owned by a corporation, give the name and address of the corporation immediately followed by the names and addresses of all stockholders owning or holding 1 percent or more of the total amount of stock. If not owned by a corporation, give the names and addresses of the individual owners. If owned by a partnership or other unincorporated firm, give its name and address as well as those of each individual owner. If the publication is published by a nonprofit organization, give its name and address.)

Full Name	Complete Mailing Address
WHOLLY OWNED SUBSIDIARY OF REED/ELSEVIER, US HOLDINGS	1600 JOHN F KENNEDY BLVD. SUITE 1800 PHILADELPHIA, PA 19103-2899

11. Known Bondholders, Mortgagees, and Other Security Holders Owning or Holding 1 Percent or More of Total Amount of Bonds, Mortgages, or Other Securities. If none, check box ▶ ☐ None

Full Name	Complete Mailing Address
N/A	

12. Tax Status (For completion by nonprofit organizations authorized to mail at nonprofit rates) (Check one)
The purpose, function, and nonprofit status of this organization and the exempt status for federal income tax purposes:
☒ Has Not Changed During Preceding 12 Months
☐ Has Changed During Preceding 12 Months (Publisher must submit explanation of change with this statement)

PS Form **3526**, July 2014 [Page 1 of 4 (see instructions page 4)] PSN: 7530-01-000-9931   PRIVACY NOTICE: See our privacy policy on www.usps.com.

---

13. Publication Title
PHYSICAL MEDICINE AND REHABILITATION CLINICS OF NORTH AMERICA

14. Issue Date for Circulation Data Below
AUGUST 2019

15. Extent and Nature of Circulation		Average No. Copies Each Issue During Preceding 12 Months	No. Copies of Single Issue Published Nearest to Filing Date
a. Total Number of Copies (Net press run)		182	192
b. Paid Circulation (By Mail and Outside the Mail)	(1) Mailed Outside-County Paid Subscriptions Stated on PS Form 3541 (Include paid distribution above nominal rate, advertiser's proof copies, and exchange copies)	85	95
	(2) Mailed In-County Paid Subscriptions Stated on PS Form 3541 (Include paid distribution above nominal rate, advertiser's proof copies, and exchange copies)	0	0
	(3) Paid Distribution Outside the Mails Including Sales Through Dealers and Carriers, Street Vendors, Counter Sales, and Other Paid Distribution Outside USPS®	40	54
	(4) Paid Distribution by Other Classes of Mail Through the USPS (e.g., First-Class Mail®)	0	0
c. Total Paid Distribution (Sum of 15b (1), (2), (3), and (4))	▶	125	149
d. Free or Nominal Rate Distribution (By Mail and Outside the Mail)	(1) Free or Nominal Rate Outside-County Copies included on PS Form 3541	42	24
	(2) Free or Nominal Rate In-County Copies Included on PS Form 3541	0	0
	(3) Free or Nominal Rate Copies Mailed at Other Classes Through the USPS (e.g., First-Class Mail)	0	0
	(4) Free or Nominal Rate Distribution Outside the Mail (Carriers or other means)	42	24
e. Total Free or Nominal Rate Distribution (Sum of 15d (1), (2), (3) and (4))	▶	42	24
f. Total Distribution (Sum of 15c and 15e)	▶	167	173
g. Copies not Distributed (See Instructions to Publishers #4 (page 43))	▶	15	19
h. Total (Sum of 15f and g)	▶	182	192
i. Percent Paid (15c divided by 15f times 100)	▶	74.85%	86.13%

* If you are claiming electronic copies, go to line 16 on page 3. If you are not claiming electronic copies, skip to line 17 on page 3.

16. Electronic Copy Circulation		Average No. Copies Each Issue During Preceding 12 Months	No. Copies of Single Issue Published Nearest to Filing Date
a. Paid Electronic Copies	▶		
b. Total Paid Print Copies (Line 15c) + Paid Electronic Copies (Line 16a)	▶		
c. Total Print Distribution (Line 15f) + Paid Electronic Copies (Line 16a)	▶		
d. Percent Paid (Both Print & Electronic Copies) (16b divided by 16c × 100)	▶		

☒ I certify that 50% of all my distributed copies (electronic and print) are paid above a nominal price.

17. Publication of Statement of Ownership
☒ If the publication is a general publication, publication of this statement is required. Will be printed
in the NOVEMBER 2019 issue of this publication.
☐ Publication not required.

18. Signature and Title of Editor, Publisher, Business Manager, or Owner
STEPHEN R. BUSHING - INVENTORY DISTRIBUTION CONTROL MANAGER

Stephen R. Bushing   Date 9/18/2019

I certify that all information furnished on this form is true and complete. I understand that anyone who furnishes false or misleading information on this form or who omits material or information requested on the form may be subject to criminal sanctions (including fines and imprisonment) and/or civil sanctions (including civil penalties).

PS Form **3526**, July 2014 (Page 3 of 4)   PRIVACY NOTICE: See our privacy policy on www.usps.com

Moving?

Make sure your subscription moves with you!

To notify us of your new address, find your **Clinics Account Number** (located on your mailing label above your name), and contact customer service at:

Email: journalscustomerservice-usa@elsevier.com

800-654-2452 (subscribers in the U.S. & Canada)
314-447-8871 (subscribers outside of the U.S. & Canada)

Fax number: 314-447-8029

Elsevier Health Sciences Division
Subscription Customer Service
3251 Riverport Lane
Maryland Heights, MO 63043

*To ensure uninterrupted delivery of your subscription, please notify us at least 4 weeks in advance of move.

Printed and bound by CPI Group (UK) Ltd, Croydon, CR0 4YY

03/10/2024

01040408-0020